COOKING FOR THE
Specific Carbohydrate
Diet

**Over 125 Easy, Healthy, and Delicious Recipes
That Are Sugar-Free, Gluten-Free, and Grain-Free**

2nd Edition

Erica Kerwien

Published by:
Ulysses Press
P.O. Box 3440
Berkeley, CA 94703
www.ulyssespress.com

ISBN: 978-1-61243-941-9
Library of Congress Catalog Number 2019905609

Printed in Korea by Artin Printing Company through Four Colour Print Group

10 9 8 7 6 5 4 3 2 1

Acquisitions Editor: Bridget Thoreson
Managing Editor: Claire Chun
Editor: Renee Rutledge
Proofreader: Barbara Schultz
Cover design: Ashley Prine
Photographs: © Erica Kerwien except page 5 yogurt © oykuozgu/shutterstock.com, page 28 chicken stock © Madeleine Steinbach/shutterstock.com, page 31 vegetables © JoannaTkaczuk/shutterstock.com, page 56 turmeric smoothie © Magdanatka/shutterstock.com, page 82 pesto © Doris Heinrichs/shutterstock.com, page 90 strawberry jam © ziashusha/shutterstock.com

IMPORTANT NOTE TO READERS
This book has been written and published strictly for informational and educational purposes only. It is not intended to serve as medical advice or to be any form of medical treatment. You should always consult your physician before altering or changing any aspect of your medical treatment and/or undertaking a diet regimen, including the guidelines as described in this book. Do not stop or change any prescription medications without the guidance and advice of your physician. Any use of the information in this book is made on the reader's good judgment after consulting with his or her physician and is the reader's sole responsibility. This book is not intended to diagnose or treat any medical condition and is not a substitute for a physician.

This book is independently authored and published and no sponsorship or endorsement of this book by, and no affiliation with, any trademarked brands or other products mentioned or pictured within is claimed or suggested. All trademarks that appear in this book belong to their respective owners and are used here for informational purposes only. The author and publisher encourage readers to patronize the quality brands and products mentioned and pictured in this book.

*To my family—for breaking bread with me nightly
and for loading and unloading the dishwasher countless times.*

Contents

Author Preface

You Are Perishable—Eat Accordingly

When my oldest child was six years old, he was misdiagnosed with scarlet fever and almost lost his life. By day three of the prescribed antibiotics his lungs were filled with fluid, he couldn't lift his body off the bathroom floor, and his fingers and toes were turning blue. I called 911 and the local fire department arrived moments later to pump his body with epinephrine and rush him to the closest emergency room. He spent the rest of the week at the hospital where he received more antibiotics, but a diagnosis was never reached. He was tested for various possible irritants and allergies but the doctors couldn't find a cause.

Over the next several years my son had a series of infections, more antibiotics, and in 2005 he was diagnosed with Crohn's disease. He was cared for by well-respected doctors in our community, and we were told there wasn't a cure or reliable treatment for Crohn's. We would have to experiment to see which pharmaceutical options best controlled the symptoms and go from there. Around this time someone told me that the Specific Carbohydrate Diet (SCD) might help my son with his Crohn's disease, yet not a single doctor mentioned a diet. In fact there was no mention of diet in the medical literature I received, and I couldn't find one on the official Crohn's and inflammatory bowel disease (IBD) websites.

Fast-forward six years. A lot has changed since I first heard about SCD. Our society is now closely scrutinizing where our food comes from and what's in it. There is a proliferation of diets that exclude processed foods, grains, dairy, and sugar, or variations on this theme. We are taking matters into our own hands: growing food ourselves, buying only from trusted sources, and finding joy in cooking at home. We also know that no single lifestyle, diet, or food pyramid fits all people. No two people are genetically the same, so it makes perfect sense that each person should eat food that works well for his or her body.

As my family began to change the way we ate, my son's health—and my family's health—improved. At the suggestion of a coworker I started a website, comfybelly.com, to track and share my recipes. My hope was that others would enjoy them and find out about SCD, and that I would learn in the process. I got all that and more. I'm so grateful that I found SCD and discovered so many other food blogs and books on SCD. But most of all, I'm grateful for Elaine Gottschall's landmark book *Breaking the Vicious Cycle*, as well as her efforts to research and publish her findings, and to reach out to so many.

The following pages are filled with new delicious recipes that work well for SCD, and I've also included some of the much-loved recipes from the *Comfy Belly* website. I hope that you can find pleasure in eating and change your life for the better, just as I and so many others have. Let food be thy medicine, or at least help the cause.

Eat well, be well,

Erica

About the Specific Carbohydrate Diet

This cookbook is filled with recipes that are grain-free, sugar-free, and gluten-free; many are dairy-free or can be made as such. The reason will be clear once you read about SCD.

A Quick History of the Specific Carbohydrate Diet (SCD)

There are so many ways to eat, ideas about eating, and reasons why people choose certain foods. The Specific Carbohydrate Diet (SCD) came from the need to heal patients who had digestive disorders and to improve digestive health.

SCD originated from a diet specifically developed by a New York physician, Dr. Sidney Haas, for his patients suffering from celiac disease. Celiac disease is an immune response to foods that contain gluten, found in many grains including wheat, barley, and rye. The disease has been documented as far back as the second century (by a Greek physician named Aretaeus of Cappadocia). Since that time, doctors have made strides to identify it and prescribe relief.

In 1955, the young daughter of Elaine Gottschall was suffering from ulcerative colitis. Elaine took a leap of faith and followed Dr. Haas's prescribed diet for her daughter. The diet healed her. Elaine went back to school to earn a master's degree in nutritional biochemistry and then shared what she'd learned in a book titled *Food and the Gut Reaction*—now known as *Breaking the Vicious Cycle: Intestinal Health Through Diet*.

Elaine's book explains the science behind SCD, so I recommend reading it to gain a full understanding of how and why this diet can work. Since the book was originally published in 1996, SCD has been used to help adults and children who have Crohn's disease, ulcerative colitis, celiac disease, cystic fibrosis, diverticulitis, irritable bowel syndrome (IBS), gluten and other food intolerances, and myriad other health issues. Elaine passed away in September 2005, but SCD continues to be used successfully, and her book has sold millions of copies.

A Bit of SCD Science

SCD guides you to eat certain kinds of carbohydrates and other foods that aid digestion and healing. The goal is to repair the injured intestinal lining, achieve a healthy balance of intestinal bacteria, improve absorption of nutrients from food, and quiet the immune system's inflammatory response that occurs with many digestive issues and diseases.

You'll notice the word "specific" in the name Specific Carbohydrate Diet. This is because you don't eliminate *all* carbohydrates, just the ones that are complex and difficult to digest. Simple carbohydrates, or *monosaccharides*, are the most basic form of a sugar and don't require digestive splitting (enzymatic digestion) in order to be absorbed into the bloodstream through the intestinal lining. Examples of foods that have monosaccharides are honey, fruit juice, and certain vegetables.

More complex carbohydrates—*disaccharides and polysaccharides*—require splitting in order to be absorbed. Disaccharides include lactose (found in cheese and milk), processed sugar (such as cane sugar), and corn syrup. Examples of foods that contain polysaccharides include rice, sweet potatoes, grains, and some vegetables.

Fiber is another beneficial component of many foods. Fiber, along with adequate amounts of water, allows food to move quickly and easily through your digestive system, sweeping and cleaning up as it goes. Fiber from fruits, nuts, and certain vegetables can be eaten when following SCD, but not the fiber from grains.

What Can I Eat?

While many diets prepare you for restrictions, SCD is nutritionally rich, delicious, and balanced, so you will likely feel grateful rather than deprived. It just takes some commitment and patience. You may feel some of the effects of this dietary change instantly, while others may be felt over a period of time, sometimes years. It's possible that SCD may not work for you and you'll need to consider that as well. Or you may need to customize SCD for your body. An elimination diet can help isolate foods that are working or not.

It's important to adhere to SCD guidelines for an extended period of time (two or more years), or indefinitely, depending on how you're doing and feeling. You'll also want to figure out which foods you don't like or can't tolerate, despite their being acceptable for SCD. Get to know your own body and what foods work for you, regardless of what SCD allows you to eat. For example, some people might find they do better when not eating nightshades, such as eggplant and tomatoes, while others will feel better if they cut dairy-based foods.

Also consider the top eight allergens: milk, eggs, tree nuts, peanuts, fish, shellfish, soy, and wheat. You'll know right away if you are allergic to a food, because you'll have an immediate reaction, such as a rash or hives, trouble breathing, swelling, or other extreme symptoms that may even threaten your life. If you don't have an allergy to a food, you may have an intolerance, which means that over time your body shows signs such as reduced energy, reduced breathing capacity, nutritional issues, and unexplained aches and pains. It's important to identify which foods aren't working for you. The easiest way to figure this out on your own is to eliminate a suspect food for a few weeks and see if you feel better.

Avoid Packaged Foods

While it's efficient to find ways to save time by using prepared and packaged food, I strongly recommend that you avoid packaged food when following SCD. Even if the ingredients on the package look like they contain only SCD-legal foods, there can be small amounts of undisclosed ingredients, such as stabilizers, or the addition of food-processing aids to keep foods fresh.

When you are following strictly SCD, many feel the only way to know for sure if a packaged food is SCD legal is to obtain a letter from the manufacturer disclosing all the ingredients. The other catch here though is that the manufacturer can change the ingredients at any time.

So, the easiest way to ensure that food is SCD compliant is to use only fresh, whole foods, or purchase prepared foods from an approved market, such as Wellbee's (see Product Sources, page 214).

Yogurt and Probiotics

Probiotics are a type of good bacteria that aid in digestion and help maintain a healthy digestive tract. By eating foods that contain probiotics and taking formulated probiotics, you can help your body "rebalance" out a build-up of bad bacteria that cause health problems. And it's a good idea to have probiotics whenever you're on prescription antibiotics, to counteract the loss of good bacteria along with the bad.

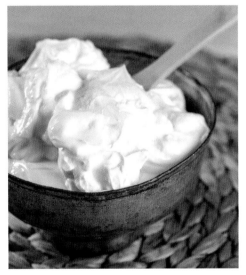

Yogurt and fermented foods will give you a good dose of probiotics, and you can get a wider variety of bacteria by supplementing your diet with a probiotic containing more strains of gut-enhancing bacteria. (See Product Sources, page 214 to find out where you can purchase SCD-compatible probiotics.)

Eating Lactose-Free

Lactose is the sugar found in dairy products such as milk, cheese, and yogurt. Because lactose is a complex sugar, it's more difficult than simple sugars to digest when you have an injured digestive system.

In general when following SCD, you can eat cheeses that have low amounts of lactose, such as Parmesan, cheddar, and Brie. I've found that it's a good idea to remove cheese and other dairy products from your diet when you're not feeling well, or at least remove any cheese that doesn't work well for you. For dairy-free milk and cream substitutions, see Basic Recipes (page 10).

Travel and Restaurant Tips

It can be challenging to find food that you can trust when you're out and about, whether it's in your own neighborhood or another country. I research restaurants and markets before I arrive in another location. Make a list of places, have back-ups, and print out maps, phone numbers, and hours of operation, and try to have a kitchen where you're staying.

When traveling by car for long distances, I find it helpful to carry a cooler for preserving food. Dried foods are also handy to have around. I'm also big on lists—lists of what you need to pack, food, and supplemental stuff you need to bring.

For air travel, don't rely on airplane food. Bring your own snacks and a bottle to fill with water. For food you'll eat over the course of a day, slip a portable dry ice pack into a soft cooler. You can also freeze some food and slip that into your goodie bag to let it defrost over travel time.

Carry water, or a water bottle that you can fill up (see Product Sources, page 214). When going to a restaurant, order or bring these foods:

◆ Foods that don't have additives (ask the waiter or manager to check on ingredients)

◆ Your own dressings (or request salt, butter, or oil to add your own seasonings)

◆ Steamed food without sauces, or food prepared with nothing other than salt, butter, or oil

◆ Simple roasted or grilled foods with only salt, butter, or oil added

School and College Tips

It was our first doctor who tipped us off to putting a plan in place at school to protect my son in case of severe illness and to ensure that he had daily support. The doctor wrote a letter explaining my son's condition and requirements and the challenges he might face.

In middle and high school, my son had a plan the school signed off on, called a 504, that allowed him access to a bathroom, food, and water at any time. The plan also made it clear that he might miss blocks of school due to illness beyond his control, and that he was to receive extended time to complete assignments when he was ill. We were lucky that the staff and teachers were accommodating, but it was good to have this plan in place just in case.

When my son was in college, he was able to work with the school to arrange special accommodations. While there's much less hand-holding in college, there are still plans in place in case of possible breaks in attendance.

The food part of living is a bit more challenging for students following SCD or any other restrictive diet. Here are some things to explore to keep your food supply up while you're away at school.

- You can use a rice steamer, slow cooker, or Instant Pot for a variety of purposes, including steaming meat, vegetables, and fruit, or for reheating and defrosting food.

- Rent or buy your own refrigerator, microwave, blender, and any other cooking appliances allowed in your dorm room, apartment, or house.

- Get to know the folks who work in your local dining halls, restaurants, and food service areas, and ask about SCD-safe foods. See if you can preorder foods in your name or arrange access to a kitchen.

- Find places to buy SCD-safe food and stores that carry brands you trust. Look into ordering food online to be delivered to your dorm room, apartment, or house.

Tips for Athletes

Athletes sometimes work themselves quite hard and try to avoid missing a workout or competition because of injury or illness. If you've watched a professional sporting event, I'm sure you've noticed an athlete getting patched up in order to get back into the game.

Sometimes, though, you just have to let it go. Slow down or take a break for a few days to give your body time to recover. If you're experiencing any discomfort or are in any way feeling less than 100 percent, any kind of athletic activity will have a greater impact on your health because your body is spending a large amount of energy just managing inflammation.

When you're working hard and have symptoms, you may be weaker, tire more easily, and not perform as you normally would. To counteract this, it's vitally important that you pay extra attention to your fluid and food intake. Take extra precautions, including drinking and eating a bit more than normal. Eating frequent, small meals (at least five a day) will help keep up your energy and stamina as well as ease the digestion process. And don't forget to get enough sleep!

That said, exercise is still quite important for keeping you as healthy as possible. When you're experiencing any symptoms, moderation is the key. A brisk walk may be all you're up for, and that's okay. The goal is to get your body moving, even if it's just for a short time.

If you're a competitive athlete, you may want to have a physical to determine if you have any vitamin or mineral deficiencies. Common deficiencies associated with digestive diseases include vitamins B6 and B12, vitamin D, and magnesium. Depending on your health care provider and the urgency of your deficiency, oral supplements or IV fluid therapy may be suggested in addition to adjusting your diet. Keep in mind that if you're on anti-inflammatory or other drug therapy, some drugs can deplete your body of vitamins and nutrients, so find out what supplements you may need to counteract this. The dosage will probably depend on your weight and the therapy, so check with your health care provider to confirm what supplements are necessary or will complement your therapy and nutrition.

Carbohydrate Intake

Whether you're a recreational or professional athlete, you probably know the importance of fluid and food intake in preparing for any athletic endeavor. Before, during, and after any high-exertion activity, you'll want to consume adequate fluids. For competitive athletes, a high-performance diet will consist of mostly carbohydrates, a moderate amount of protein, and a smaller amount of fat.

You may be somewhat concerned about how SCD fits in with your athletic life, especially if your source of energy before changing your diet was complex carbohydrates such as potatoes and pasta. You'll just be changing your sources of carbohydrates, not reducing your intake of carbohydrates. When following SCD, the carbohydrates are mostly simple sugars such as those in fruits, vegetables, nuts, seeds, honey, yogurt, and cheese.

It's important to eat foods in combination to keep your body from absorbing carbohydrates too quickly. Adding protein and a small amount of fat to a meal prevents the carbohydrates from being absorbed too fast. You want to prevent that feeling of high and low sugar levels in your bloodstream. You'll experience steady energy levels during times of exertion from a balance of carbohydrates, protein, and fat. You may find that your body uses the foods you eat more efficiently, since they stay around longer—especially proteins and fats.

A steady stream of carbohydrates, plus protein, is essential to maintaining healthy blood glucose levels. Eat before, during, and after any exercise that lasts more than an hour in order to maintain your energy level. It's also important to replenish your body with carbohydrates and fluids within an hour of heavy exertion so that your body can begin replenishing electrolytes and glucose, repair tissues, and rebalance fluids.

Workout Food List

The following foods will help you get enough carbohydrates, protein, fat, and fluids to perform your best. It's easiest to eat in small spurts so as not to overwhelm your digestive system. Small bites throughout the day work well.

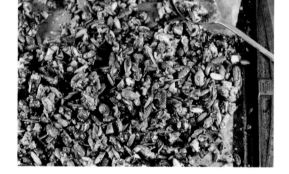

- Pickles and pickled salads—excellent sources of electrolytes

- Fresh fruits such as bananas, apples, berries, oranges, pears

- Applesauce, pear sauce, cheese sticks, crackers, granola (page 178), and even ketchup (page 80) to give you quick energy for recovery

- Breakfast Cookies (page 204), quick breads, and fruit and nut bars

- Steamed vegetables in Classic Marinara Sauce (page 78) or salad dressing, veggie-based soups, and salted broth

- Frittatas, egg scrambles with veggies, pesto, or fruit (apple-egg scrambles are my favorite)
- Sports drinks (page 34) with small amounts of salt plus fruit or honey, or both
- Lightly salted vegetable juices, gazpacho (page 73), or smoothies with a bit of salt added
- Fruit in yogurt (page 20) or fruit and cheese sandwiches, such as Apple Cheddar Panino (page 94); cheese; and pickles

High-Performance Tips

I've been an athlete all my life, and while I don't have autoimmune or digestive issues, just a quick walk with the dog helps me feel better and recover faster when I've been sick. Walking gets your entire body working, including your digestive system.

If you're an athlete on a special diet such as SCD, here are some things to keep in mind. This list is good for all athletes, but I have a special affinity for athletes persevering in the face of challenging conditions. I've helped my son keep playing sports in some of the most challenging conditions, and as a result he has learned how to care for himself, both physically and mentally.

- Always get enough rest, and sleep on a regular schedule.
- Moderate how much exercise you do on a daily basis according to your health at the moment.
- Eat enough carbohydrates, protein, and fat in combination to avoid low blood glucose.
- Drink, drink, drink—electrolytes, juice, water, soups, broths.
- Try to eat small meals or snacks every couple of hours or so.
- Carry extra snacks to eat before, during, and after any athletic endeavor.
- Eat within 60 minutes of any high-exertion activity.
- Have fun, and don't be too hard on yourself! You're working extra hard to stay healthy, and that's no small feat.

Basic Recipes

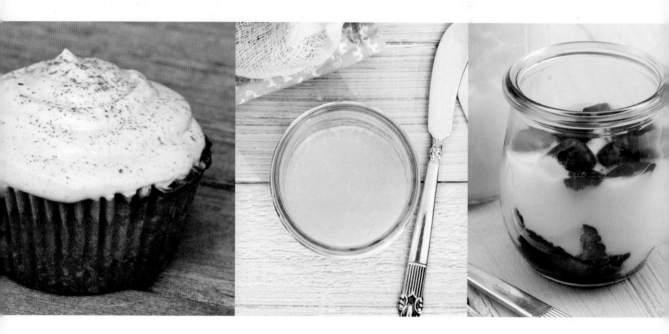

Here is a collection of basic recipes and techniques that can be used on their own or as part of other recipes, including many in this book. I use some of these recipes on a weekly basis. You'll find both dairy-based and dairy-free recipes, as well as both vegetarian and meat-based recipes.

Soaked Nuts, Seeds, and Beans

Soaking nuts, seeds, and beans (legumes) is a great idea, and just requires a bit of planning—mostly to allow enough soaking time. Most seeds, nuts, and beans (and grains, by the way) are coated with enzyme inhibitors to prevent them from sprouting (growing) prematurely. Soaking initiates enzyme activity, making these foods easier to digest and their nutrients more available and easily absorbable. Many nuts also taste better after they've been soaked, especially walnuts and almonds. This is because any tannins, dust, and residue from the skins is released into the soaking water, leaving the soaked nut with a smoother, buttery flavor.

Quick Tips

◆ You can store soaked (and drained) nuts and seeds in the refrigerator for a day or so if you're not quite ready to use them.

◆ Make sure you're soaking the raw, unsalted, and unprocessed form of seed, nut, or bean.

◆ Some legumes, such as red lentils, don't need soaking.

In general, you want to soak nuts and seeds until they're softened. For SCD, soak all beans overnight. The chart on page 12 will help guide you—in general, the denser the nut, seed, or bean, the longer the soaking time. Here's how to proceed:

1. Remove nuts or seeds from their shells, if they have them.

2. Fill a container with about double the amount of water as nuts, seeds, or beans to be soaked. If you are soaking 2 cups of almonds, for example, soak them in 4 cups of water. Many nuts, seeds, and beans will expand while soaking.

3. Soak for anywhere from 15 minutes to overnight. The goal is to soak until the nuts, seeds, or beans start to soften. The necessary soaking time varies—check the chart on page 12 for estimated soaking time for some types.

4. Rinse and drain the nuts, seeds, or beans until the water is clear. Let them drain fully and then they're ready to use in a recipe. You can also dry them in a dehydrator if you want them completely dry.

Nut/Seed/Bean (raw)	Soak Time
Almonds	8 to 12 hours
Black beans	Overnight
Brazil nuts	Don't soak
Cashews	4 to 8 hours
Hazelnuts	Don't soak
Lentils	Overnight
Macadamias	Don't soak
Dried peas	Most need 12 hours; follow the directions that come with the peas
Peanuts	8 hours
Pecans	8 hours
Pepitas (pumpkin seeds)	8 hours
Pine nuts	Don't soak
Pistachios	Don't soak
Sesame seeds	8 hours
Sunflower seeds	2 hours
Walnuts	4 hours

Almond Milk (and Other Nut Milks)

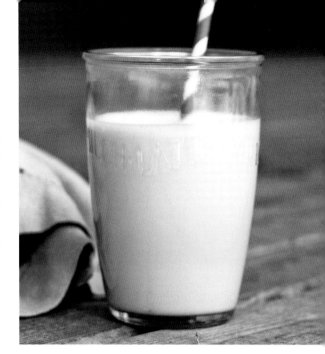

Almond milk is my favorite dairy-free milk. It can be used in soups, baking, tea, smoothies, or just to drink on its own. I make my own almond milk because it's difficult to find almond milk that works for SCD due to the additives in most brands. To change it up, this recipe also works with other nuts, such as macadamias, Brazil nuts, and hazelnuts. Or try a mixture of nuts, or use seeds, if you prefer.

As almond milk sits in the refrigerator, it will separate. Just whisk or shake it up again before drinking or using it in a recipe. Besides the water and nuts, you'll also want a nut milk bag (see Product Sources, page 214), or use several layers of cheesecloth. Leggings and tights work, too! The almond pulp that remains can be used to make crackers (see Parmesan Crackers, page 46, and Almond Saltine Crackers, page 48).

Makes 2 (1-cup) servings

1 cup raw almonds

2 cups water

1. Place the almonds in a bowl and cover them with water to soak overnight.

2. Drain and rinse the almonds and place them in a high-speed blender. Add 2 cups of water to the almonds and blend until completely ground up; I blend mine for about 1 minute.

3. Drain the almond milk through a nut milk bag (or several layers of cheesecloth) into a pitcher or bowl.

4. Store in the refrigerator for up to several days.

Nutrition per serving: *30 calories, 3 g fat, 1 g carbohydrate, 1 g fiber, 1 g protein*

Sweet Almond Milk

The only difference between this and the straight-up almond milk above is that you add ½ teaspoon vanilla extract and 2 dates to give it a subtle sweetness. Or you could just stir in ½ teaspoon vanilla extract and 2 teaspoons honey. This milk is good by itself at any time of day, and in smoothies and tea—as well as for cookie dunking.

Almond SCD Yogurt

Homemade yogurt tastes nothing like the store-bought versions I've had. Even if you don't eat dairy-free, this is a really nice, mellow yogurt with a subtly sweet flavor. While this recipe is a bit more detailed than making regular yogurt, it's totally worth it for the taste, in my humble opinion.

You can make this using any nut milk, including hazelnut and cashew milk—see my recipes for nut milks in this chapter. Since almond milk doesn't contain lactose, you'll need to add some honey so the starter bacteria have something to munch on (culture). Or you can use a sweet milk as the base. I don't culture this yogurt as long as for dairy-based yogurts; you can culture it for more than 4 hours, but there's no pressing need to do so, since it contains no lactose.

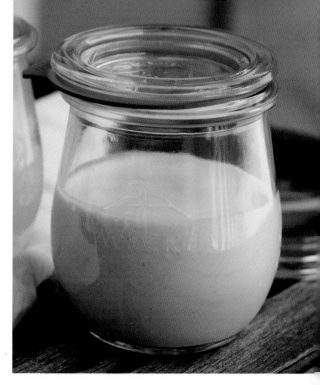

You'll notice that I add gelatin to thicken the yogurt. If you don't add the gelatin, the yogurt will have more of a thick liquid consistency. That works well if you're using it to make a probiotic drink or a milkshake. Otherwise I suggest including the gelatin for a thicker, yogurt-like texture. You may have to experiment a bit to obtain the thickness you like, and it will also depend somewhat on the gelatin brand. In general, I add less gelatin than most manufacturers call for, because I don't want the yogurt to completely gel. If your almond yogurt is too thick, you can blend in more almond milk, fruit juice, or cooked fruit. You can easily double or triple this recipe.

Makes 2 (1-cup) servings

2 cups almond milk

1 tablespoon honey

½ teaspoon unsweetened powdered gelatin (see Product Sources, page 214)

yogurt starter (see Product Sources, page 214, for dairy-free starters; I use about ⅛ teaspoon dairy-free starter, but check the manufacturer's directions for the suggested amount)

1. Place the almond milk and honey in a saucepan over low to medium heat. Heat for about 5 minutes, or until the honey is dissolved and the liquid is steaming and has begun to bubble. Stir occasionally to prevent separation. You want the temperature of the milk to be around 180°F/80°C. The milk may thicken a bit.

2. Remove from the heat and let cool to room temperature.

3. Whisk the gelatin into the cooled milk until blended. Add the yogurt starter and blend until dissolved and evenly distributed.

4. Place the milk in a yogurt maker, or set in a warm environment, such as a dehydrator, that stays between 100°F/38°C and 110°F/43°C. Culture for at least 4 hours (or follow the yogurt starter directions).

5. Cover and refrigerate for at least 1 hour. You can store the yogurt in the refrigerator for up to a week.

Nutrition per serving: *92 calories, 3 g fat, 17 g carbohydrate, 1 g fiber, 1 g protein*

Coconut Milk

My favorite thing about this recipe is that I can have dairy-free coconut milk in just a few minutes. While you can soak the shredded coconut for 2 hours, I usually just soak it in hot water for a few minutes and move on to the next step. It's up to you. Soaking longer gets you a slightly thicker, more flavorful cup of milk, but the shortcut is nothing to sneeze at, especially if you have a really good high-speed blender.

Coconut milk can be used in soups and smoothies and for baking. I prefer to make it from shredded coconut, because it's easy and the coconut is additive free. I sometimes wonder what's in a can of coconut milk and how long it's been sitting on the shelf. In a pinch, though, I'll use a can that doesn't have any additives (see Product Sources, page 214), but read the label carefully—most canned coconut milk has one or more additives.

As coconut milk sits in the refrigerator, it will separate. Just whisk or shake it up again before drinking it or using it in a recipe.

Makes 2 (1-cup) servings

1 cup unsweetened shredded coconut (see Product Sources, page 214)

2 cups water

1. Combine the shredded coconut and water in a blender container and let soak for about 2 hours. Or, if you're short on time, soak the coconut in hot water (about the temperature of hot tap water) for a few minutes and move on to the next step.

2. Blend the coconut and water in a high-speed blender on the highest speed.

3. Strain the coconut milk through a nut milk bag or several layers of cheesecloth into a pitcher or bowl. Store in the refrigerator for up to several days.

Nutrition per serving: *45 calories, 4 g fat, 1 g carbohydrate, 0 g fiber, 0 g protein*

Tips

◆ Coconut flakes will work also.

◆ If you have a fresh coconut, add the water and flesh to a high-speed blender or food processor. Blend it until broken down into a slurry and then follow the directions for soaking and then draining the milk in step 3.

◆ Feel free to add a pinch of salt and a teaspoon or two of honey to flavor the milk.

◆ This sweetened version of the basic recipe above is equally delicious on its own or in smoothies or other recipes. When you blend the soaked coconut, simply add 2 pitted Medjool dates or about 2 tablespoons honey, and 1 teaspoon vanilla extract. Then strain the milk through a nut milk bag or a few layers of cheesecloth set on top of a fine-mesh strainer.

Cashew Milk

Cashew milk is dairy-free milk that can be used for baking or cooking, or you can drink it on its own, hot or cold. Sweetening it up a bit adds to the goodness. While you don't have to soak the cashews (see page 11 for directions) before making the milk, it does tend to come out a bit creamier when you do. You'll need a high-speed blender to get the milk as creamy as possible. As cashew milk sits in the refrigerator, it will separate—just whisk it again before serving it or using it in a recipe.

Makes 4 (1-cup) servings

    1 cup raw cashews

    4 cups water

1. Place the cashews and water in a high-speed blender and blend until the nuts are completely ground up.

2. The milk will separate after several hours and can then be blended again or mixed by hand.

3. Cover and store in the refrigerator. It will last for several days in the refrigerator.

> **Nutrition per serving:** *25 calories, 2 g fat, 1 g carbohydrate, 0 g fiber, 1 g protein*

Tips

◆ Adding natural sweetener and flavoring to cashew milk makes it into a sweet treat. Follow the basic recipe but add 2 pitted Medjool dates or about 2 tablespoons honey, and 1 teaspoon vanilla.

◆ I store cashews and other nuts in my refrigerator to extend their shelf life to about 6 months.

◆ If the milk is too thick for your taste, add more water.

Sweet Cashew Cream

This dairy-free whipped cream can be flavored to suit your taste or the recipe you're adding it to. For example, add a little lemon or orange juice for a tangy version to use with lemon-flavored baked goods. Or add cinnamon, nutmeg, or other spices. You can store the soaked and drained cashews in the refrigerator for a day or two until you're ready to use them.

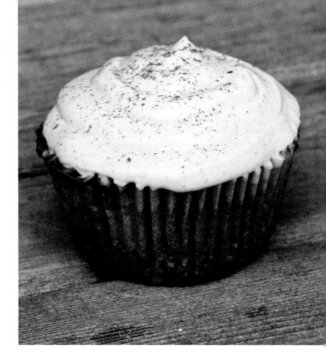

Makes 8 (¼-cup) servings

1 cup raw cashews

3 cups water, for soaking

¼ cup fruit juice or coconut water, or more as needed

2 Medjool dates, pitted (or substitute 2 tablespoons of honey)

½ teaspoon vanilla extract

pinch of salt (or to taste)

pinch of ground cinnamon, to serve (optional)

1. Soak the cashews in about 3 cups of water for at least 4 hours, or overnight.

2. Drain the cashews and then rinse them with water and drain again.

3. Combine all the ingredients except for the cinnamon in a high-speed blender and process for about 1 minute, or until creamy. Add more juice or coconut water if the mixture seems too thick or isn't blending well. (You can use a food processor or a regular blender, but it will take longer.)

4. Cover and store in the refrigerator for up to a few weeks. Serve with a pinch of ground cinnamon, if using.

> **Nutrition per serving:** *100 calories, 6 g fat, 9 g carbohydrate, 1 g fiber, 3 g protein*

Modify SCD for Your Body

If you need to be dairy-free, find dairy-free substitutes. Find the foods that work best for your body and fit into the list of SCD-compatible foods. You may think that doesn't leave you much to eat, but you may just need to take some time to learn about flavors and how various foods complement each other.

Sour Cashew Cream

Here's a dairy-free version of sour cream that can be used in many recipes and as a topping for soups, nachos, and other savory dishes. It helps to have a high-speed blender or food processor when whipping it up, but you can also use a regular blender—just keep it running for a while to make sure the nut pieces are all ground up. You can use sour cashew cream in most recipes that call for yogurt, such as many of the dips and sauces in this book. Use your imagination to add flavors that will enhance a dish—lime and chili powder, for example. For a dairy-based, lactose-free sour cream, see the recipe for crème fraîche, page 24.

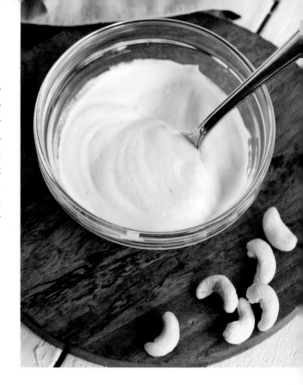

Makes 4 (¼-cup) servings

1 cup raw cashews

3 cups water, for soaking

2 teaspoons fresh lemon juice

salt, to taste

3 tablespoons water, or more as needed

1. Soak the cashews in about 3 cups of water for at least 4 hours, or overnight. Drain, rinse with water, and drain again.

2. Place the cashews, lemon juice, and salt in a high-speed blender; add 3 tablespoons of water. Blend until the mixture until is creamy and smooth, about 1 minute; add more water if needed. (If you're using a regular blender or food processor, it will take longer.)

3. Store in the refrigerator, sealed airtight, for up to about a week.

Nutrition per serving: *171 calories, 12 g fat, 11 g carbohydrate, 1 g fiber, 5 g protein*

Simple Cashew Cream

Here's a simple, versatile cashew cream that can be used whenever you want to add a cream base to a recipe. Try it with Creamed Spinach (page 144) or dairy-free Mushroom Soup (page 75), or any time you want to mimic the flavor and consistency of dairy-based cream.

Makes 8 (2-cup) servings

1 cup raw cashews

3 cups hot water

1. Soak the cashews in 3 cups of hot water for 20 minutes.

2. Drain the cashews, reserving 1 cup of the soaking water.

3. Add the reserved water and cashews to a food processor or blender and process until the mixture is creamy.

> **Nutrition per serving:** *80 calories, 6 g fat, 4 g carbohydrate, 1 g fiber, 3 g protein*

Buy in Bulk and Freeze

Buy more than you need and freeze the rest. When they're in season, I buy loads of strawberries, blueberries, and other fruits or vegetables that can easily be frozen for later. You can buy flour in bulk and freeze or refrigerate it for later, too. Nuts and nut oils tend to spoil quickly, so I store those in the refrigerator if I know I won't be plowing through them right away.

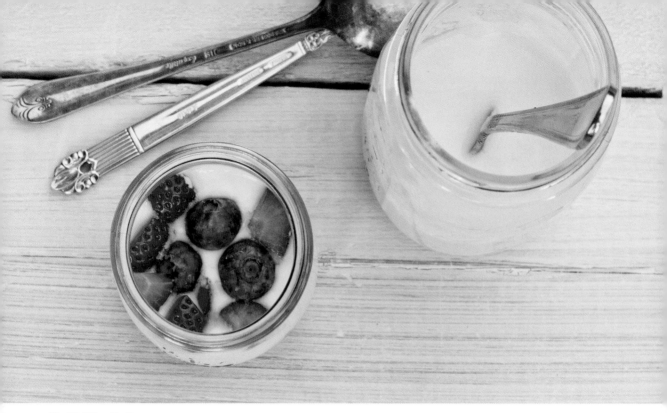

SCD Yogurt

Homemade yogurt is easy to make and so economical. It's also a good thing for intestinal healing because it contains good bacteria for your digestive system. If you can't have dairy or simply don't like yogurt, I suggest finding a probiotic as a source of good bacteria (see Product Sources, page 214).

There are just two requirements for SCD Yogurt: it must be cultured for 24 hours (to ensure that the lactose is removed), and it must contain beneficial bacteria that will help the gut heal. The bacteria come from the starter you add to the milk—either yogurt or a yogurt starter. In either case, the recommended cultures are lactobacillus bulgaricus, L. acidophilus, and S. thermophilus. In Elaine Gottschall's book, *Breaking the Vicious Cycle*, she recommends that you avoid bifidus because it has been known to cause digestive issues.

While you can use yogurt from previous batches as a starter, I prefer not to; it never turns out quite as well, in my experience. But it works in a pinch. For more on yogurt starter, see Product Sources, page 214.

Makes 8 (½-cup) servings

4 cups milk (cow's, goat's, or sheep's milk)

about 1 tablespoon yogurt starter

1. Pour the milk into a saucepan, place it on low to medium heat and bring the milk to a steady simmer. When the milk reaches about 180°F/90°C, remove it from the heat and let cool to room temperature.

2. Pour about ¼ cup of the cooled milk into a sterile container that has a cover. Add the yogurt starter and stir to blend well. Pour in the rest of the milk and blend well.

3. Place in a yogurt maker or other warm environment, between 100°F/38°C and 110°F/43°C, for 24 hours.

4. After 24 hours, refrigerate the yogurt until you're ready to use it. It will keep for a few weeks in the refrigerator.

> **Nutrition per serving:** *35 calories, 2 g fat, 3 g carbohydrate, 2 g protein, 0 g fiber*

Dripped SCD Yogurt

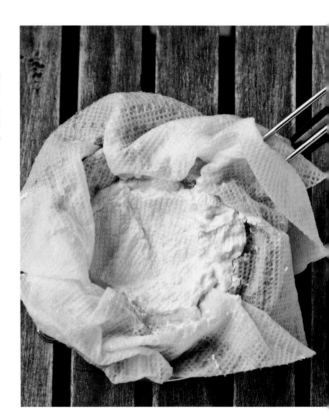

Dripped yogurt—also called strained or Greek yogurt—is thick yogurt that's had a lot of its moisture dripped out of it. I use dripped yogurt whenever a recipe calls for Greek yogurt, or when I want to reduce the amount of moisture added to a recipe. It also makes an excellent substitute for cream cheese or farmer's cheese (pot cheese).

1. Set a mesh strainer or colander over a bowl to catch the dripping liquid from the yogurt (whey). Line the strainer with cheesecloth, a coffee filter, or a few sheets of paper towels.

2. Place the yogurt in the lined strainer. You don't need to refrigerate the dripping yogurt, but I tend to do so in case I don't use it right away. Let it drip for at least 30 minutes, or up to at least 6 hours for cream cheese consistency.

3. Once you have cream cheese, you can add salt and herbs to create a tasty dip or a spread for sandwiches.

Herbed Cream Cheese

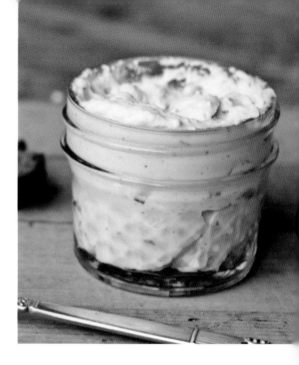

This recipe uses dripped (Greek) yogurt. The longer you drip the yogurt, the firmer your cream cheese will be. I try to let it go for at least a day to get really thick cream cheese. In the end, you have a creamy, lactose-free cheese spread that can be flavored to your liking.

You don't need to heavily season this cheese to enjoy it; I just think the seasoning adds a lot of dimension to the rich creaminess of the cheese. If you use goat's-milk yogurt, your cream cheese will become a creamy herbed goat cheese.

Makes 4 (¼-cup) servings

2 cups SCD Yogurt (page 20)

1 tablespoon minced fresh parsley

½ teaspoon dried dill weed

¼ teaspoon salt

¼ teaspoon garlic powder

¼ teaspoon onion powder

1. Drip the yogurt for 24 hours, following the Dripped SCD Yogurt directions on page 21.

2. Blend the resulting cream cheese in a bowl with all the remaining ingredients, using a whisk or fork, until the mixture is well blended and creamy.

3. Cover and store in the refrigerator for up to a few weeks.

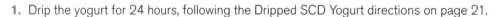

Nutrition per serving: *35 calories, 2 g fat, 3 g carbohydrate, 2 g protein, 0 g fiber*

Tip

♦ You can try a variety of seasonings, using either fresh or dried herbs. If you're using dried herbs, you'll need less than for fresh herbs. If you'd normally use 1 tablespoon fresh thyme, for example, then you'll only need 1 teaspoon dried thyme.

Clarified Butter and Ghee

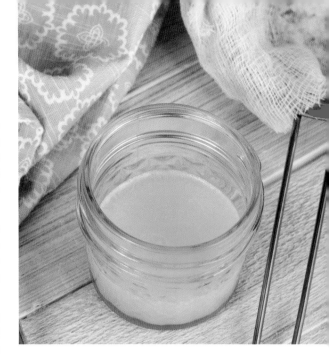

Clarified butter is butter from which the water and milk solids have been removed. This is done both for flavor and to raise the butter's smoking point so that it can be used at high temperatures, such as when sautéing, roasting, or grilling. It has the added side benefit of removing milk solids, which may be difficult for some to digest or tolerate.

Ghee is just like clarified butter, except that the milk solids are browned before being removed. The result is that ghee has a slightly stronger, nuttier flavor than clarified butter. To make ghee, follow the directions for clarified butter and keep heating it until the milk solids turn brown.

Clarified butter and ghee will stay fresh for at least a month at room temperature, or at least four months in the refrigerator. I use clarified butter for frying and sautéing. I make big batches and leave a jar out at room temperature for cooking, while the rest is stored in the refrigerator. When I'm getting low, I just pull out a new jar and bring it to room temperature before I use it.

Serving size is 1 tablespoon

unsalted butter

1. Melt the butter in a saucepan over medium heat until it begins to simmer. (This is the water escaping.)

2. Simmer slowly until the milk solids have separated to the bottom, some foam sits on top, and the clear yellow clarified butter sits in the middle. This takes about 10 minutes. If you're making ghee, continue heating until the milk solids on the bottom of the saucepan have turned brown (to about 250°F/120°C)— but don't let them burn. Don't stir the butter.

3. Use a fine-mesh strainer lined with cheesecloth to strain the butter (or ghee) into a jar or other container. The milk solids and excess foam will separate out and the clarified butter will drip into the jar.

4. Store at room temperature for up to about a month, or keep in the refrigerator for a few months.

> **Nutrition per serving:** *102 calories, 12 g fat, 0 g carbohydrate, 0 g protein, 0 g fiber*

Crème Fraîche (Sour Cream)

I used to buy cultured sour cream for soups, dressings, and dips. Now I much prefer this creamy cultured crème fraîche. Traditional crème fraîche is made with buttermilk, but this version is made with the same yogurt starter you use to make SCD-style lactose-free yogurt. Use it in recipes that call for sour cream, crème fraîche, or extra-creamy yogurt. It's also great as a tangy substitute for whipped cream.

Try flavoring this with lemon, herbs, and spices to create creamy dips and dressings. My favorite variation has a pinch of salt, some minced green herbs, crushed fresh garlic, lemon juice, and a drizzle of olive oil.

Makes 8 (¼-cup) servings

2 cups heavy cream

yogurt starter (see Product Sources, page 214)

1. Pour the cream into a saucepan, place on a low to medium heat, bring it to a simmer, and then remove from the heat and let cool to room temperature.

2. Pour some of the cooled cream into a sterile container that has a lid. Add the yogurt starter according to the manufacturer's instructions and stir to blend well. Add the rest of the cream and blend well.

3. Place the container in a yogurt maker, or other warm environment, between 100°F/38°C and 110°F/43°C, for 24 hours.

4. After 24 hours, place the cream in the refrigerator until you're ready to use it.

> **Nutrition per serving:** *205 calories, 22 g fat, 2 g carbohydrate, 1 g protein, 0 g fiber*

In the Beginning

Start with broths and steamed veggies, and go easy on fruit and dairy. Raw foods are challenging to digest, so steer clear of salads for a while. And when you have a setback, return to the basics that make you feel good.

Ricotta Cheese (Dairy-Free)

Here's an easy recipe for dairy-free ricotta cheese using cashews. You can use it in a variety of recipes that call for ricotta cheese, and you can bake with it.

Makes 1 cup (16 tablespoons)

1 cup raw cashews

3 cups water, for soaking

2 tablespoons lemon juice

½ teaspoon salt

1. Soak the cashews in about 3 cups of water for at least 6 hours, or overnight; you can also soak for 1 hour in boiling water. Drain, rinse with water, and drain again.

2. Place the cashews, lemon juice, and salt in a high-speed blender. Blend until the mixture until is creamy and smooth, about 1 minute; add more water if needed. (If you're using a regular blender or food processor, it will take longer.) Use a spatula to scrape down the sides in between processing.

3. Store in the refrigerator, sealed airtight, for up to about a week.

> **Nutrition per tablespoon:** *40 calories, 3 g fat, 2 g carbohydrate, 1 g protein, 0 g fiber*

Whipped Cream

You can whip yogurt cream the same way you'd whip heavy cream—it just has a tangier taste. It's like having whipped yogurt. You can add flavor with vanilla extract, honey, or cinnamon, or just use it on its own. Yogurt cream goes great with granola, strawberries, and other fruit; on top of muffins; and as a filling for crêpes.

Makes 8 (¼-cup) servings

  2 cups crème fraîche (page 24)

  1 tablespoon honey, or to taste

  ¼ teaspoon vanilla extract

1. Place all the ingredients in a bowl and whip for several minutes, or until the mixture becomes lighter and forms soft peaks. I use my stand mixer with the whip attachment, but you can use a hand or standing mixer, or a whisk.

2. Cover and store in the refrigerator for up to a few days.

> **Nutrition per serving:** *205 calories, 22 g fat, 2 g carbohydrate, 1 g protein, 0 g fiber*

Nut Butter

Nut butters such as almond and cashew are easy to make—and most of the time the homemade version will cost you less than a jar of the premade version. To make nut butter, you just process the nuts in a high-speed blender or food processor until they go from nuts to flour to butter. It can take a few minutes, depending on the nuts and whether you've soaked them.

You can make butter from cashews, hazelnuts, sunflower seeds, or other nuts and seeds—and peanuts, of course (a legume). If you like your nut butter salted, just add a bit of sea salt, or you can add honey, cinnamon, or vanilla. You get the idea. Yes. It's that simple. The nutrition information varies depending on the nuts you use; the figures below are based on almond butter.

Makes 8 (¼-cup) servings

  2 cups raw or roasted nuts (if you're using raw nuts, soaking is optional; see page 11)

1. Place the nuts in the container of a food processor or high-speed blender.

2. Blend for about 5 to 10 minutes, depending on the nut and whether it has been soaked.

3. Store nut butter in a sealed container for about a month, or in the refrigerator for several months.

> **Nutrition per serving:** *27 calories, 3 g fat, 1 g carbohydrate, 1 g protein, 0 g fiber*

Nut Flour

Many of the baked goodies in this book are made with blanched almond flour, but you can try other nut flours, such as walnut and cashew. In case you're wondering what types of nut flour are out there, here's a quick primer.

The nuts can be raw or roasted. Each will yield a different flavor. *Almond meal* is ground-up raw almonds with their skins on. *Blanched almond flour* is a ground-up raw almonds that have had the skins removed. Unless otherwise noted, recipes in this book use finely ground blanched almond flour. This is the nut flour I bake with the most, because it produces a texture that I like. That being said, many of my bread and muffin recipes will also work with almond meal as well as other nut flours, though they'll taste a bit different than if made with blanched almond flour.

Some nut flours (such as cashew) are easy to make, while others require a bit more preparation if you don't want the nut skins in the flour. Almonds are the prime example. For blanched almond flour, you can buy almonds with the skins off (blanched), use diced or sliced almonds, or purchase blanched almond flour (see Product Sources, page 214). Some recipes work well without blanching, but if you want to emulate baked goodies made with all-purpose flour, you'll want the skins off.

Makes 8 (¼-cup) servings

2 cups raw or roasted nuts or seeds

Place the nuts in the container of a high-speed blender or food processor and pulse until you have fine grains of flour. Be careful not to pulse the flour too much or you'll end up with nut or seed butter. Another option is to use a coffee grinder to grind the nuts, grinding small batches at a time.

Nutrition per serving: *40 calories, 4 g fat, 2 g carbohydrate, 2 g protein, 1 g fiber*

Tips

- Not all ground-nut flours have the same fineness in grind. If you'd like your flour to be finer than it is, place it in a food processor and grind it to a finer texture.
- If you're using almonds, remove the skins to produce blanched almond flour.
- If you're soaking the nuts, dry them completely before grinding them.

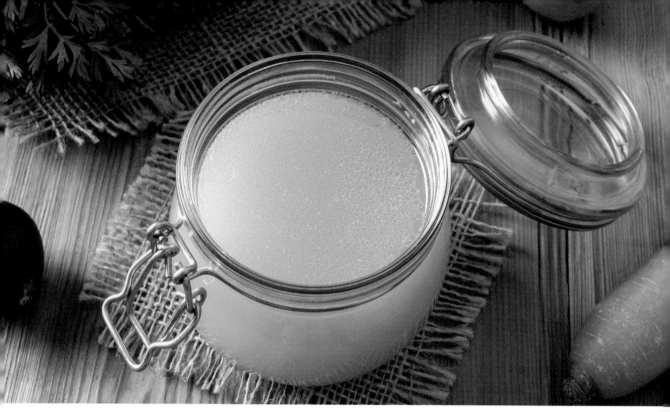

Chicken Broth

Chicken broth is so soothing to the body and soul. Serve this broth on its own, or use it to build nutritious soups, stews, pureed vegetables, and other recipes that call for savory liquids. And bone broth is an excellent way to replenish your body with fluids and nutrients.

I freeze chicken broth in 2-cup portions because this size is easy to add to recipes or make a big bowl of soup. You may want to freeze smaller amounts in an ice cube tray for adding a bit of flavor to a marinade or to a soup or sauce. Label your containers and keep them in the freezer for up to a few months. When freezing the broth in a jar or other container, leave some space at the top to allow for expansion as the liquid freezes.

Makes 8 (1-cup) servings

1 chicken carcass, whole chicken pieces, 1 whole chicken, or chicken bones

8 cups water (or enough to cover most of the chicken)

4 cups (approximately) of diced vegetables or vegetable scraps (such as carrots, celery, leeks, and onions; avoid cabbage, which tends to make the broth bitter)

chopped herbs, herb scraps, or other seasonings (such as thyme, parsley, garlic, chives, green onions, kosher or sea salt, pepper; optional)

1 tablespoon apple cider vinegar (optional)

1. Add the chicken carcass or pieces to a stockpot filled with about 8 cups of water.

2. Add diced vegetables and any seasonings you're using. You can add cut carrots (which make the broth sweet), leeks, celery, onions, herbs, and salt and pepper to taste (if you want it pre-seasoned). Add the vinegar, if using.

3. Let simmer for at least 3 hours on a low heat, covered.

4. Remove from the heat, let cool, and strain the liquid through a fine-mesh strainer.

5. Discard everything but the broth. Cover and store the broth in the refrigerator for up to about a week, or keep in the freezer for several months.

> **Nutrition per serving:** *50 calories, 1 g fat, 0 g carbohydrate, 10 g protein, 0 g fiber*

Tips

♦ Add about 1 tablespoon vinegar when cooking the broth to release more calcium from the bones, soften them, and produce a better soup gel.

♦ If you're using a roasted chicken from the store (usually rotisserie style, ready to eat) and it has extra seasonings, remove the skin to avoid over-seasoning the stock. I suggest purchasing the most natural version of the store-bought roast chicken that you can, to avoid additives and unwanted seasonings.

♦ This is a quick way to recover the pan drippings from roasted chicken for use as chicken broth. It comes in handy when you need some chicken broth in a hurry to make gravy and pureed vegetables. Add the pan drippings from a roasted chicken or chicken pieces to a pot with about 3 cups water (about 1 cup for each tablespoon of drippings). Place the pot over medium heat and bring to a steady simmer, and continue simmering for 10 minutes. Turn off the heat, let cool for a bit, and strain the liquid through a mesh strainer. Cover and store in the refrigerator for about a week or in the freezer for a few months. Makes about 4 cups.

♦ You can use an Instant Pot (or other pressure cooker) to save time—you'll get a rich broth that is ready in just 1 hour. Add all the ingredients to your pressure cooker, fill with enough water to cover the vegetables and chicken, and cook on high pressure for 45 to 60 minutes.

♦ For a richer broth, keep the skin on the chicken.

♦ You can also add ginger, black pepper, bay leaves, and garlic to the broth. I don't add salt while cooking because I prefer to add it once I'm cooking or making soup from the broth. If you are using leftover chicken, it may already have seasoning and salt added.

Beef Broth

Bone broths are great for warming your body and boosting your immune system and overall health. They're rich in minerals such as calcium and phosphorus, soaked from the bone and marrow. In addition, the joint tissues contain collagen and other supplemental compounds that are good for bone and tissue health.

For this recipe, the beef bones are roasted before the long simmer to preserve and bring out their best flavor. While you might be tempted to skip this step, take the extra time to roast the bones and the veggies in order to produce an exceptionally flavored broth.

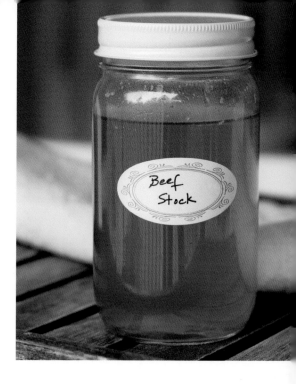

Makes 8 (1-cup) servings

2 pounds meaty beef bones (from grass-fed cows, if possible)

2 large carrots, cut into a few large chunks

1 large onion, cut into a few large chunks

about 8 cups water

sweet vegetable scraps: celery, carrot, leek, onion, garlic

1 tablespoon apple cider vinegar (or other vinegar or lemon juice)

salt and pepper

1. Preheat your oven to 400°F/200°C.

2. Place the beef bones, carrots, and onions on a rimmed baking sheet and roast for 30 minutes.

3. Let the roasted bones and veggies cool for a bit and then place them in a large stockpot or slow cooker with about 8 cups of water and the vegetable scraps, vinegar, and salt and pepper to taste.

4. Cover and simmer on a low heat for about 5 hours.

5. Let cool and then strain the beef broth to remove all veggies, bones, meat, and residual scraps, using a fine-mesh strainer.

6. Cover and refrigerate for a few hours or overnight and then skim the fat off the top of the beef broth. Store in the refrigerator for several days, or freeze for later use.

Nutrition per serving: *10 calories, 0 g fat, 1 g carbohydrate, 0 g fiber, 2 g protein*

Vegetable Broth

Vegetable broth is a great way to capture the minerals and vitamins in a variety of vegetables, as well as enhance the flavor of another recipe. It also can serve as the basis for just about any soup. The classic recipe for vegetable broth is to simmer sweet vegetables such as carrots, onions, leeks, and garlic for a few hours. Vegetables you *don't* want to use in a broth include beets, broccoli, kale, lettuce, and squash. Most of these don't add flavor to the broth, and vegetables that are part of the brassica family (such as cabbages, cauliflower, and broccoli) will add a bitter taste. You can make frozen vegetable bouillon by whirling raw vegetables in a food processor until they're the consistency of pesto, then freezing in small containers, bags, or ice cube trays.

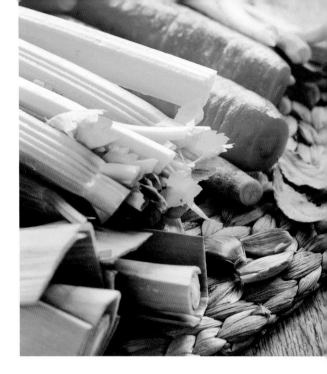

Makes 6 (1-cup) servings

> 1 tablespoon ghee (page 23) or butter
>
> 1 leek, cut into thin rings
>
> 1 carrot, peeled and coarsely chopped
>
> 1 celery stalk, chopped
>
> 1 medium garlic clove
>
> 1 small bunch parsley, chopped
>
> salt and pepper, to taste
>
> water to cover the veggies (at least 6 cups)

1. Place all the ingredients in a large saucepan over a medium heat and bring to a boil.

2. Reduce the heat to low and simmer for an hour or so, until all the vegetables are tender.

3. Strain the liquid through a fine-mesh strainer, discarding the vegetable pieces. Cover and store in the refrigerator for a few days, or freeze for up to several months.

Nutrition per serving: *10 calories, 0 g fat, 2 g carbohydrate, 0 g fiber, 0 g protein*

Mushroom Broth

Great in soups and sauces, this is my favorite broth because its dark, earthy flavor is based solely on vegetables and seasonings. I use cremini mushrooms.

Makes 10 (1-cup) servings

1 large yellow onion, trimmed, peeled, and chopped

1 pound mushrooms or mushroom stems

1 carrot, cut into coins, or a cup of carrot trimmings

2 cloves garlic

1 tablespoon red wine vinegar

1 teaspoon salt

10 cups water (or enough to cover all the ingredients in the pot)

1. Add all the ingredients to a large pot and bring to a boil.

2. Reduce the heat and simmer for 1 to 2 hours.

3. Strain the broth and discard the solids. Store the broth in the refrigerator for a few days or freeze for a few months.

> **Nutrition per serving:** *14 calories, 0 g fat, 2 g carbohydrate, 1 g fiber, 1 g protein*

Tips

◆ Freeze your vegetable scraps and when you're ready to make broth, just pull them out and toss them in the pot.

◆ You can cook the broth in an Instant Pot (or other pressure cooker) for 40 minutes.

◆ You can slow-cook the broth on low for 8 hours.

◆ You can replace red wine vinegar with a legal version of balsamic vinegar (no sugar added).

◆ Herbs and seasonings to add include black pepper, parsley, thyme, and bay leaf.

Filtered Water

I like drinking water that has been filtered using a carbon filter. There are several ways to do this, but no matter which method you choose, I think you'll notice that the flavor is improved. What you won't notice are the residual chemicals that have been removed. This depends on your water source, but most tap water contains chlorine and fluoride along with small amounts of other chemicals that you don't want to ingest on a regular basis.

Here are some ways to filter your water:

- Charcoal-filtered water bottle (see Product Sources, page 214)
- Refrigerator water dispenser with water filter insert
- Filtered water bottle stored in your refrigerator
- Filter attachment on your water faucet
- Filter attachment at your home's main water source

Hydrate

Having enough water in your body at all times is essential to your health. Water carries nutrients throughout the body, eliminates waste, lubricates joints, and cushions organs. Drink lots of water, broth, and electrolytes to keep everything moving, replenish water lost due to diarrhea, flush out toxins, and make it easier to digest your food. While you don't want to drink too much water, finding a happy balance is important. I prefer filtered water because it removes excess residue found in tap water, including chlorine, pesticides, and prescription drug residue increasingly found in water sources. One of my favorite portable sources of filtered water is a charcoal-filtered water bottle (see Product Sources, page 214).

Sports Drinks (Electrolytes)

Just about any fruit drink or smoothie can be turned into an electrolyte with the addition of a natural source of salt. Two ingredients to add to an electrolyte are a simple carbohydrate, such as citrus fruit or fruit juice, and a source of sodium and possibly potassium, as from iodized sea salt.

Here are two basic electrolytes, one using fruit juice and the other using both dairy-free milk and coconut water. The fruit juice drink might be acidic, depending on the juice you use; that might cause irritation for some, in which case you can choose a less acidic juice, such as apple or grape juice.

Coconut water is a natural electrolyte and sweetener that contributes essential minerals, including potassium, calcium, and magnesium. If you don't have coconut water, you can substitute water and 2 tablespoons honey.

Fruit Juice Electrolyte

Makes 4 (1-cup) servings

>   3 cups water
>
>   1 cup fresh orange juice (or other juice, such as apple, grape, or a combination of lemon and a sweet juice)
>
>   ½ teaspoon iodized salt

In a container that has a cap or cover, mix all the ingredients together until the salt is dissolved. Cover and store in the refrigerator for up to a few weeks.

> **Nutrition per serving:** *28 calories, 0 g fat, 6 g carbohydrate, 0 g fiber, 0 g protein*

Dairy-Free Milk Electrolyte

Makes 4 (1-cup) servings

>   2 cups dairy-free milk (almond, coconut, or other)
>
>   2 cups coconut water (or 2 cups water with 2 tablespoons honey)

Mix all the ingredients together in a bottle or other container until the salt is dissolved. Cover and store in the refrigerator for up to about a week. Shake as needed to blend again.

> **Nutrition per serving:** *15 calories, 1 g fat, 1 g carbohydrate, 1 g fiber, 1 g protein*

Tomato Sauce

You can use tomato juice to make tomato sauce. According to the book *Breaking the Vicious Cycle,* tomato juice from a can is allowed if salt is the only addition. This means you don't need confirmation with the manufacturer that there are no additives in their canned version. This is a very flexible recipe, so feel free to adjust the seasonings to your liking.

Makes 4 (6-tablespoon) servings

3 cloves garlic, minced

1 small yellow onion, diced

2 teaspoons dried oregano or basil

1 carrot, peeled and grated

½ teaspoon salt

1 (48-ounce) can tomato juice

1 tablespoon honey

1. Add all the ingredients except the honey into a large stockpot.

2. Simmer uncovered over low heat for 1½ hours, or until the sauce has thickened enough.

3. Add the honey and stir with a spoon.

4. Cool a bit before serving. Store in the refrigerator for a few days or freeze for a few months.

Nutrition per serving: *76 calories, 0 g fat, 18 g carbohydrate, 3 g fiber, 2 g protein*

Tomato Paste

Like the Tomato Sauce recipe above, you can use tomato juice to make tomato paste. Make sure it doesn't have any other additives other than salt. It won't be as thick as store-bought tomato paste, but it's a great base for sauces, the ketchup recipe on page 80, and the barbecue sauce recipe on page 36.

Makes 4 (¼-cup) servings

1 (48-ounce) can tomato juice

1. Pour the tomato juice into a large saucepan over medium heat and bring to a boil.

2. Reduce the heat to low and simmer uncovered for 1 to 1½ hours, stirring occasionally, until the sauce is reduced to the thickness you desire. Store in the refrigerator for a few weeks or freeze for a few months.

Nutrition per serving: *65 calories, 0 g fat, 2 g fiber, 2 g protein*

Mayonnaise

Homemade mayonnaise is easy to make with a food processor—you'll just need a few pantry staples. You generally want to use a mild-flavored oil as your choice will affect the flavor of the mayonnaise; I prefer sunflower oil because it has little to no flavor. Olive and avocado oils impart more flavor to the mayonnaise. In a pinch, you can substitute vinegar for lemon juice. And feel free to use your favorite mustard as well.

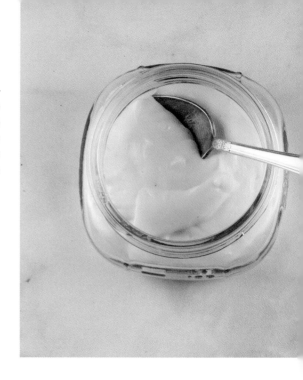

Makes 1 cup (18 servings)

1 large egg

1 teaspoon lemon juice

1 teaspoon Dijon mustard

drizzle of honey (optional)

1 cup oil

1. In a food processor or blender, add the egg, lemon juice, mustard, and honey, if using. Blend on high while slowly drizzling the oil into the mixture.

2. Store covered in the refrigerator for a few weeks.

Nutrition per serving: *111 calories, 12 g fat, 0 g carbohydrate, 0 g fiber, 0 g protein*

Barbecue Sauce

This is a quick and easy recipe for barbecue sauce. Use it when serving ribs or any other grilled or roasted entrées. Store in the refrigerator for a few weeks, or freeze leftovers for a few months.

Makes 8 (¼-cup) servings

⅔ cup Tomato Paste (page 35)

⅔ cup white vinegar

½ cup honey

½ teaspoon smoked paprika

¼ teaspoon salt

1. Add all the ingredients to a saucepan and stir to blend.

2. Place the saucepan on a stovetop over low heat and simmer the sauce for 5 to 10 minutes.

3. Cool to room temperature and serve.

Nutrition per serving: *118 calories, 0 g fat, 28 g carbohydrate, 1 g fiber, 1 g protein*

Fruit Juice Gelatin

Use your favorite fruit juice for this simple recipe for Jell-O fans. Apple, grape, raspberry, or apple cider works well but remember to choose a 100 percent pure fruit juice that has no added sugar or other ingredients. I recommend avoiding acidic juices such as orange and pineapple because these don't set well. If the fruit juice is not very sweet, add a little honey.

Makes 4 (½-cup) servings

¼ cup cool water

1 envelope or 1 tablespoon unflavored gelatin

¼ cup boiling water

1 tablespoon honey, optional

1½ cups fruit juice

1. Place ¼ cup cold water in a bowl and sprinkle in the gelatin. Let soften for a few minutes.

2. Add the boiling water and honey, if using, then stir to combine.

3. Add the fruit juice and stir to combine.

4. Cover the bowl and refrigerate for a few hours, or until it's set.

Nutrition per serving: *50 calories, 0.1 g fat, 11 g carbohydrate, 0.1 g fiber, 1.6 g protein*

Tip

♦ Rub oil on the inside of your mold so the gelatin slips out easily once it's set.

Small Bites and Snacks

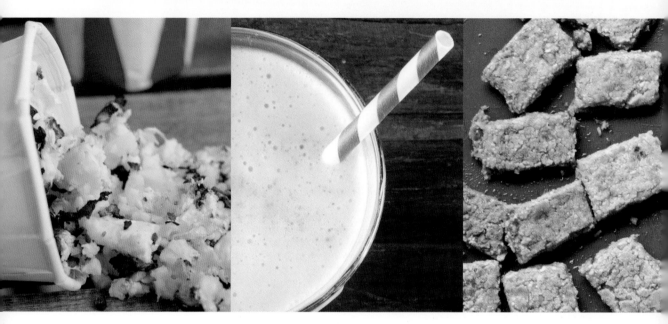

The flavor-packed recipes on the following pages can be shared as appetizers or packed as snacks. Snacking is always fun, and you'll find a variety of snacks here to satisfy you when you're craving some quick and easy bites.

Cherry Pecan Bars

Here's a date-nut-fruit bar that's great to have around for quick energy and nutrition after a run or bike ride, or just as a midday snack. You'll need a food processor or high-speed blender to whip up these bars, but that's all you'll need besides the nutritious ingredients. You can substitute other dried fruits or nuts for what's listed, which will change the taste a bit depending on the ingredients.

Be sure to use dried fruit and nuts that have no added sugar, honey, oil, or other additives. Dried cranberries, for example, tend to have oil and apple juice added to make them tastier; I love that for some recipes, but the added oil makes these bars greasy.

Makes 8 bars

½ cup dried tart cherries

½ cup whole pitted Medjool or other dates

1 cup raw or roasted pecans (I use raw, but both work)

⅛ teaspoon salt, or to taste

1. Place all the ingredients in the bowl of a food processor or high-speed blender. Pulse until the mixture is ground well and can be pressed into bars (usually a minute or so).

2. Press the ground mixture into a square (about 9 x 9-inch) or rectangular pan or baking dish, flattening it to cut into bars.

3. Store covered at room temperature for about a week, or in the refrigerator for a few weeks. I individually wrap my bars in waxed paper so they're easy to grab for on-the-go snacking.

> **Nutrition per bar:** *128 calories, 10 g fat, 10 g carbohydrate, 2 g fiber, 1 g protein*

Limit Almond Flour

While almonds are a rich source of minerals, healthy fat, fiber, and protein, don't try to fill up on treats made from almond flour. Also try other nut flours and coconut flour when you're baking. Focusing on vegetables, fish, poultry, and a small amount of fruit will be healthier and easier on your body.

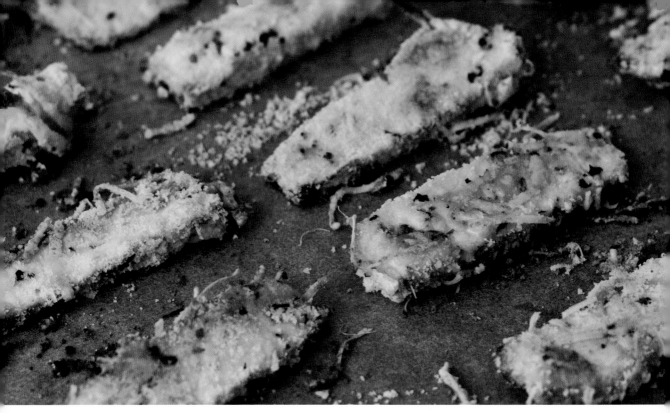

Zucchini Sticks

I love the taste of almond flour, cheese, and egg coating on fish, chicken, and veggies such as these zucchini sticks. They're terrific with many kinds of dips and dressings, including Caramelized Onion Dip (page 86) and Ranch Dressing (page 83). For more ideas, see the Sauces, Jams, and Dips chapter (page 77). Zucchini tend to contain a lot of moisture that gets released when they're cooked. To reduce the water content before using them in a recipe, you can let them sweat out some of the moisture in a colander for 15 minutes or more (as instructed below). This recipe also works well without the almond flour; replace flour with the equivalent amount of Parmesan cheese, grated or shredded.

Makes 4 (2-stick) servings

4 medium zucchini, peeled and cut into 3-inch sticks

1 ¼ teaspoons salt, divided

¼ cup blanched almond flour

1 teaspoon dried oregano

1 teaspoon dried basil

½ cup grated Parmesan cheese

½ cup shredded Parmesan cheese

2 eggs, lightly beaten

dip, for serving

1. Place the zucchini sticks in a colander (or on a paper towel) and sprinkle with 1 teaspoon salt. Toss to coat well with the salt. Let sit for at least 15 minutes.

2. Preheat your oven to 425°F/220°C. Line a baking sheet with parchment paper or other nonstick material.

3. In a bowl, blend together the almond flour, remaining ¼ teaspoon salt, oregano, basil, and grated and shredded Parmesan. Whisk the eggs in a separate bowl.

4. Dry the zucchini sticks using a paper towel or cloth. Coat each stick with egg, dredge in the cheese-flour mixture, and place on the prepared baking sheet.

5. Bake for about 10 minutes, or until browned. Let cool for a few minutes and then serve with a dip.

6. Store leftovers in a closed container in the refrigerator for several days, or freeze for up to a month or so. Reheat the frozen zucchini sticks at 325°F/175°C for 6 to 8 minutes.

Nutrition per serving: *482 calories, 36 g fat, 12 g carbohydrate, 3 g fiber, 30 g protein*

Candied Nuts

Sweet nuts are a quick, high-protein snack that travels well. Use any blend of nuts and seeds that you like; my favorite mix is walnuts, pumpkin seeds, and sesame seeds. If you do combine nuts and seeds, make sure your choices take around the same amount of time in the oven to avoid uneven baking.

Makes 8 (¼-cup) servings

2 cup walnuts or nuts of your choice

½ teaspoon cinnamon

½ teaspoon nutmeg

2 tablespoons unsalted butter, melted

6 tablespoons honey

pinch of salt

1. Preheat the oven to 325°F/165°C.

2. Line a baking sheet with parchment paper or a nonstick baking mat.

3. In a bowl, mix all the ingredients together until the nuts are well-coated.

4. Spread the nuts across the baking sheet and bake for 15 minutes, or until they start to brown.

5. Cool for 10 minutes, or until dry.

6. Store sealed in a container for a few days or in the refrigerator for a few weeks.

Nutrition per serving: *216 calories, 15 g fat, 20 g carbohydrate, 4 g fiber, 5 g protein*

Tips

- Feel free to vary the seasonings and spices you add. If you like spicy nuts, add some black pepper, curry and ginger powder, or even a small amount of cayenne pepper.

- To make this dairy-free, substitute oil for butter.

- For a salty-sweet treat, add ¼ teaspoon salt.

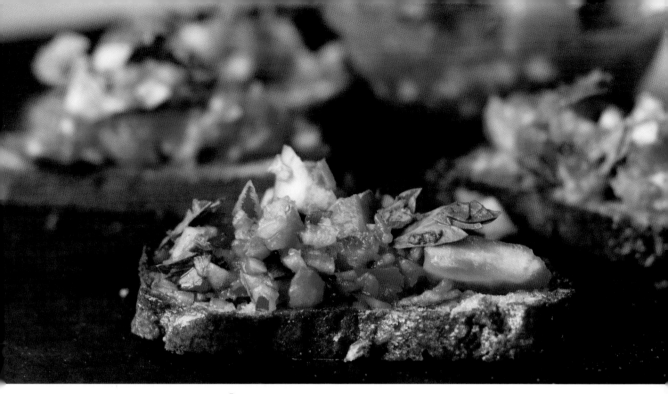

Tomato Bruschetta

You can make this bruschetta mixture any time of the year, but it's especially tasty during the summer months when you have a good batch of sweet tomatoes. Cherry tomatoes, when in season, are especially good in this recipe.

As far as bread, use any recipe you prefer. I love toasting up several slices of garlic toast and then topping them with this. It also goes well alongside grilled fish, chicken, and vegetables, or as a topping for a pizza or flatbread (see Pizza Crust, page 119).

Makes 8 servings

4 large plum tomatoes (about 1½ pounds), diced into large pieces

¼ cup diced onion (optional)

2 medium garlic cloves

1 tablespoon chopped fresh basil (or fresh oregano or parsley)

1 teaspoon red wine vinegar

2 tablespoons olive oil

½ teaspoon salt

Garlic Toasts (page 120), to serve (optional)

1. Place the tomatoes, onion (if using), and garlic in a food processor and gently pulse until the pieces are finely chopped. Alternatively, you can chop these ingredients by hand.

2. Transfer the tomato mixture to a bowl and blend in the remaining ingredients.

3. Let sit for an hour or so if time permits. Serve with Garlic Toasts or with a meal.

Nutrition per slice: *50 calories, 3 g fat, 4 g carbohydrate, 1 g fiber, 1 g protein*

Grilled Cheese Croutons

Grilled cheese is the ultimate comfort food for many. Once you've made the grilled cheese sandwich, you can decide to stop there, but cutting these into croutons gives you a wonderful topping for soup, stew, or chili. See the Breads, Biscuits, and Crêpes chapter (page 91) for some excellent bread options.

Makes 12 croutons

½ tablespoon butter, ghee (page 23), or cooking oil

your favorite cheese, shredded or sliced (cheddar, Havarti, and Swiss cheese are good options)

2 slices of bread from this book, or other SCD bread

1. Warm a skillet over medium heat. Melt the butter or ghee, or heat the oil in the skillet.

2. Create a cheese sandwich by placing the cheese between the bread slices. Set the sandwich in the heated skillet and grill on each side for about 5 minutes, or until the cheese begins to melt and the bread is toasted.

3. Let cool for a moment, slice into croutons, and serve.

Nutrition per crouton: *37 calories, 2 g fat, 3 g carbohydrate, 0 g fiber, 2 g protein*

Balancing Your Diet

Try not to get caught up in balancing your diet based on standard food pyramids—they don't apply here. Balanced nutrition does matter, though. You may be forgoing some things by not having grains or cereals, so you'll need to balance that out another way, which I find is essential for healing and general mental health. Seek out a health professional to find out what vitamins and minerals you may need boosted a bit. Vitamin D, B12, and folic acid tend to be low in folks who have digestive issues.

Parmesan Crisps

This quick and simple snack contains just a single ingredient—Parmesan cheese. Or two ingredients, if you want to sprinkle some dried oregano or basil on top of each cracker. If you don't have Parmesan cheese, another aged hard cheese will also work.

Makes 22 crisps

4 ounces Parmesan cheese, shredded

dried oregano or basil (optional)

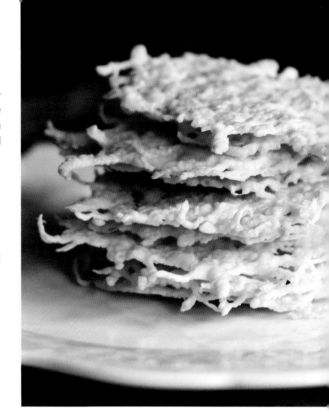

1. Preheat your oven to 350°F/175°C. Line two baking sheets with parchment paper or nonstick baking mats.

2. Drop about 1 tablespoon shredded Parmesan cheese at a time onto the lined cookie sheet. If you want the crisps to be thick in the center, pile the cheese in a mound and it will spread as it bakes. If you want them to be crunchy and lacy, spread the cheese out evenly. Sprinkle with dried oregano or basil, if you wish.

3. Bake for 6 minutes, or until the tops are starting to brown.

4. Let cool for a few minutes and then crunch away. Store at room temperature in a sealed container for a few days, or in the refrigerator for a few weeks.

Nutrition per crisp: *22 calories, 1 g fat, 0 g carbohydrate, 2 g protein*

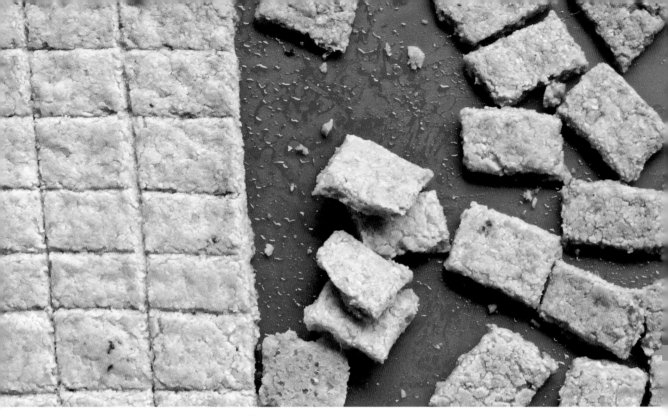

Parmesan Crackers

Use these as either croutons or crackers, or crumble crackers to use as a crunchy topping for other dishes. I like to keep it simple, seasoning-wise, but this recipe could stand up to many seasoning modifications and additions. My favorite is just garlic powder and salt, and maybe some dried thyme or oregano. You can substitute almond pulp for the almond flour (see Almond Milk, page 13), in which case you won't need the cold water to hold the dough together; the moisture in the pulp will probably be enough.

Makes 30 crackers

1 ½ cups grated Parmesan cheese (about 6.5 ounces)

1 ½ cups blanched almond flour

¼ teaspoon salt

½ teaspoon garlic powder

½ teaspoon dried thyme or oregano (optional)

2 to 3 tablespoons cold water

1. Preheat your oven to 350°F/175°C.

2. Using a food processor or blender, pulse together all the ingredients except for the water.

3. Add the cold water, a bit at a time, until the mixture is holding together well enough to work into a ball.

4. Separate into 2 balls of dough and place each on a nonstick baking mat, parchment paper, or other nonstick surface that can be transferred to a baking sheet. Roll each ball into a sheet of dough about ⅛ inch thick, taking time to roll it evenly into a rectangular shape (since the outer edges will tend to bake faster).

5. Using a pizza cutter or soft-edged knife if you are using silicone mats, gently score the dough into squares for crackers or croutons. Lift the mats or parchment paper onto two baking sheets.

6. Bake for 25 minutes, or until the crackers or croutons are browned—the darker they are, the crunchier they'll be. If the crackers in the center of the baking sheets aren't fully crunchy, turn off the oven, remove the outer crackers to cooling racks, and leave the soft crackers in the oven for another 5 minutes.

7. Let cool, break the sheets into crackers, and store in a sealed container for several weeks.

Nutrition per cracker: *48 calories, 4 g fat, 1 g carbohydrate, 1 g fiber, 3 g protein*

Almond Saltine Crackers

This recipe can be the basis for more elaborate crackers you may be craving, but if what you want is a simple, slightly salty cracker, then just stay with the basics. You can dip these crackers in a variety of things—soups, cheese spreads, creamy dips, and preserves. Or make Herbed Cream Cheese (page 22) and Cured Salmon (page 170), and have a little party.

If you feel like dressing up these crackers before they go in the oven, stir some seeds or seasoning into the dough or sprinkle some on top before you slide it into the oven. Give a gentle press to make things stick, or lightly brush the top with an egg white wash before you do the sprinkling.

Makes 30 crackers

2 cups blanched almond flour

½ teaspoon salt, plus more for sprinkling

1 large egg

1 tablespoon olive oil or unsalted softened or melted butter

1. Preheat your oven to 350°F/175°C.

2. Combine the almond flour and ½ teaspoon salt in a bowl and blend well. Blend in the egg and oil or butter. Shape the mixture into 2 balls.

3. Place each dough ball on a nonstick silicone baking mat. Place a piece of parchment paper (or another mat) over the ball and roll the dough into a thin layer, about ⅛ inch thick, taking care to roll it evenly into a rectangular shape (since the outer edges tend to bake faster).

4. Score into cracker shapes using a pizza cutter or soft knife if you're using a silicone mat. Sprinkle salt lightly across the cracker sheet.

5. Bake for about 15 minutes, or until the crackers start to brown lightly. If the crackers in the center aren't yet fully crunchy, remove the outer crackers to a cooling rack, turn off the oven, and leave the soft crackers in for another 5 minutes.

6. Let cool for about 15 minutes and then break apart into crackers. Store the crackers in a sealed container at room temperature for several weeks.

> **Nutrition per cracker:** *43 calories, 4 g fat, 1 g carbohydrate, 1 g fiber, 2 g protein*

Salt and Pepper Crackers

Here's a simple, dairy-free cracker that can be spiced up or down to your liking. Be sure to use blanched almond flour and not almond meal. Almond meal is ground almonds with the skins still intact, whereas blanched almond flour has the skins removed. When finely ground, blanched almond flour gives baked goods a texture that is similar to all-purpose flour without the carbs!

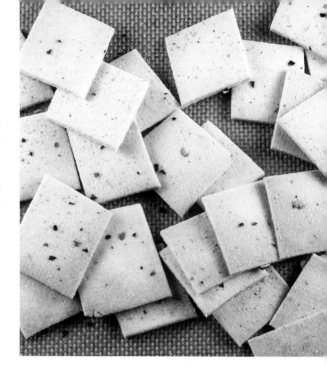

2 cups blanched almond flour

1 large egg

½ teaspoon salt, plus more to taste

½ teaspoon red or black pepper, plus more to taste

Makes 40 crackers

1. Preheat your oven to 350°F/175°C.

2. In a food processor, add the flour, egg, and ½ teaspoon of salt, and pulse until a ball forms.

3. Place the dough ball on a nonstick silicone baking mat. Place a piece of parchment paper (or another mat) over the ball and roll the dough into a thin layer, about ⅛ inch thick or thinner, taking care to roll it evenly into a rectangular shape (since the outer edges tend to bake faster). The thinner the dough the crisper the cracker.

4. Transfer the bottom paper with the crackers to a baking sheet and lightly sprinkle the dough with more salt and pepper.

5. Use a knife or pizza cutter to divide the dough into cracker squares. Lightly sprinkle salt and pepper across the crackers.

6. Bake for 20 minutes or until the crackers begin to lightly brown.

7. Let cool for about 15 minutes and serve. Store the crackers in a sealed container at room temperature for several weeks.

Nutrition per cracker: *34 calories, 3 g fat, 1 g carbohydrate, 1 g fiber, 1 g protein*

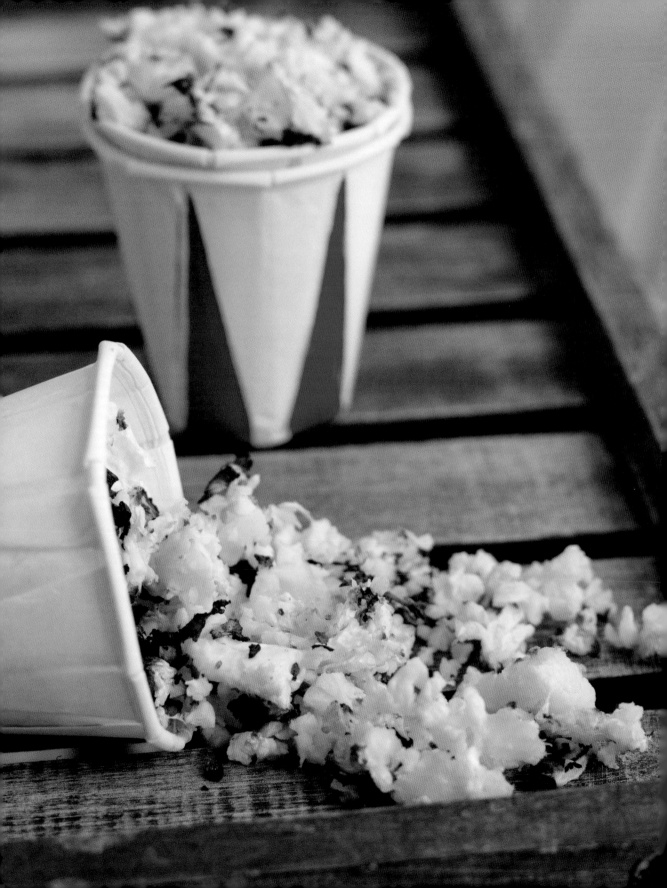

Cauliflower Popcorn

This is a light treat, sort of like popcorn in intent and flavor, with the texture on the crisped edges of the cauliflower bits. This isn't going to fill a big bowl like its namesake, but it's divine in its own way. Feel free to play around with toppings, such as cumin, chili powder, flavored salts, or turmeric to give the "popcorn" a deep yellow coloring.

I try not to use too much oil, so that the cauliflower crisps without burning too much. If you don't like the cauliflower bits this dry, add a bit more oil or ghee. Or top the popcorn with melted butter once it's out of the oven.

Makes 4 (¾-cup) servings

2 large cauliflower heads

1 tablespoon high-heat oil or melted ghee (page 23), or as desired

¼ teaspoon sea salt

1. Preheat your oven to 425°F/220°C. Line two rimmed baking sheets with parchment paper or nonstick baking mats.

2. Using a knife, dice the cauliflower heads into pieces about the size of popped popcorn kernels, all about the same size so they'll roast fairly evenly.

3. Mix the cauliflower, oil, and salt in a bowl until the pieces are well-coated.

4. Spread them out on the prepared baking sheets.

5. Bake for 15 minutes, or until all the cauliflower is crisped around the edges. Let cool for a moment before removing from the baking sheets and serve immediately.

Nutrition per serving: *103 calories, 4 g fat, 15 g carbohydrate, 6 g fiber, 6 g protein*

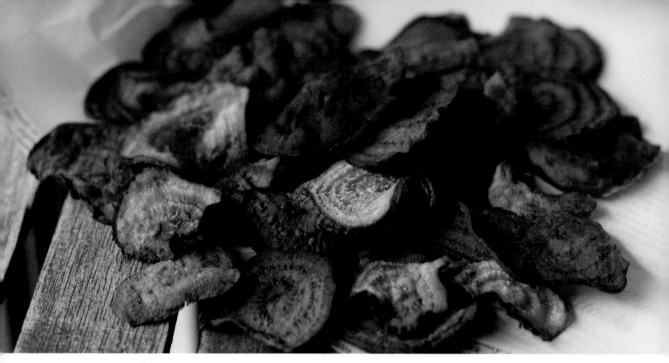

Beet Chips

These chips have a slightly sweet flavor and a nice, light crunch. A mandolin works well for slicing the beets evenly and thinly, but it isn't absolutely necessary. If you have a slicing attachment for your food processor, that also works well. I use a paring knife, and that does the job pretty well, but it takes awhile.

If the chips become soft, just place them in the oven for 5 minutes or so at 350°F/175°C to crisp them again.

Makes 4 servings

> 4 large beets—red, gold, striped (Chioggia), or any combination
>
> 1 to 2 teaspoons olive oil (or other cooking oil)
>
> sea salt, to taste

1. Preheat your oven to 350°F/175°C. Line two baking sheets with parchment paper or nonstick baking mats.

2. Peel the beets and slice them very thin—about $1/16$-inch thickness.

3. Combine the beet slices and olive oil in a bowl and toss well to coat evenly.

4. Place the beet slices on the prepared baking sheets and sprinkle lightly with salt. Bake for about 30 minutes or until the beets are curling around the edges.

5. Let cool for a few minutes so the beet chips become crunchy, and then serve. Store in a sealed container for a few days.

Nutrition per serving: *50 calories, 2 g fat, 8 g carbohydrate, 2 g fiber, 1 g protein*

Herbed Goat Cheese

Traditionally, goat's milk is heated and then curdled with lemon juice to produce goat cheese. To make some that is SCD legal, you'll need to first make Dripped SCD Yogurt using goat's milk (or you can purchase SCD-legal dripped yogurt farmer's cheese).

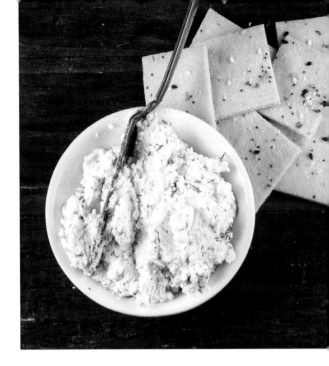

Makes 8 (2-tablespoon) servings

1 cup goat's milk Dripped SCD Yogurt (page 21)

1 tablespoon fresh dill, basil, mint, or other herb

1. Combine the cheese and herbs with a spatula. Sprinkle herbs on top as well.

2. Cover and store in the refrigerator for several days.

> **Nutrition per serving:** *103 calories, 8 g fat, 0 g carbohydrate, 0 g fiber, 6 g protein*

Tips

♦ Instead of herbs, add a topping. My favorite is caramelized onions: Finely chop 1 red onion then sauté in olive oil until the onion is soft and transparent.

♦ For a rich pop of flavor, try Parsley and Spinach Pesto (page 81) or dairy-free Basil Walnut Pesto (page 82).

♦ Combine flavoring with seeds, such as an everything seasoning, which has sesame seeds, poppy seeds, garlic, onion, and salt.

Cauliflower Hummus

You can make hummus using white beans that are SCD legal (I have a recipe on my site for just that). When you're looking for a lighter take on this portable snack, use roasted cauliflower.

Makes 8 (¼-cup) servings

1 large cauliflower head, trimmed and cut into florets

4 cloves garlic, chopped

½ teaspoon salt

2 tablespoons tahini

3 tablespoons fresh lemon juice

2 tablespoons olive oil, plus more to blend and serve

pinch of sweet paprika, to serve

vegetables (such as carrots and peppers) and crackers, to serve

1. Preheat the oven to 450°F.

2. Prepare a baking sheet with parchment paper or a nonstick baking mat.

3. In a large bowl, add the cauliflower, garlic, 2 tablespoons olive oil, and salt, and mix well.

4. Spread the mixture in a single layer on the prepared baking sheet and bake for 20 minutes or until the tips of the florets begin to brown.

5. Place the roasted cauliflower, tahini, and lemon juice in the food processor and blend until smooth.

6. Add additional olive oil to make it smooth and pulse a few times until just blended. Add more salt and lemon juice to taste.

7. Place the hummus in a bowl, drizzle with additional olive oil, and sprinkle with paprika. Serve with vegetables and crackers.

Nutrition per serving: *55 calories, 4 g fat, 5 g carbohydrate, 2 g fiber, 2 g protein*

Tips

♦ Use another teaspoon of lemon juice for added zing (this is how I like it!).

♦ If you find the hummus too thick, add water 1 tablespoon at a time until it reaches the desired consistency.

♦ You can also add ½ teaspoon cumin.

♦ If you're not eating raw, steam or roast the vegetables being served with the hummus. Carrots, broccoli, zucchini, and onions are all great options.

Tzatziki

Tzatziki is a refreshing Greek dip made with strained yogurt, cucumbers, garlic, and lemon. It goes well with crackers, raw or roasted vegetables, and spicy or salty dishes as a cooling counterpart. Pair this cool dip with the Almond Saltine Crackers (page 48), Peri Peri Chicken (page 154), or Jamaican Jerk Chicken (page 151).

Makes 8 (¼-cup) servings

1 small cucumber, peeled and finely chopped

1 tablespoon salt

1½ cups Dripped SCD yogurt (page 21)

2 cloves garlic, minced

1 tablespoon lemon juice

1 tablespoon olive oil

1 tablespoon fresh dill, minced

1. Add the cucumbers and salt to a colander and place in the sink to sweat for 10 minutes. Rinse and set aside.

2. In a large bowl, add the yogurt, garlic, lemon juice, oil, dill, and cucumbers, and stir to combine.

3. Store in the refrigerator up to a week.

> **Nutrition per serving:** *30 calories, 2 g fat, 2 g carbohydrate, 0 g fiber, 2 g protein*

Tips

◆ You can substitute white vinegar for lemon juice.

◆ I recommend seedless or Persian cucumbers.

◆ To make this dairy-free use dairy-free Ranch Dressing (page 84) in place of the yogurt.

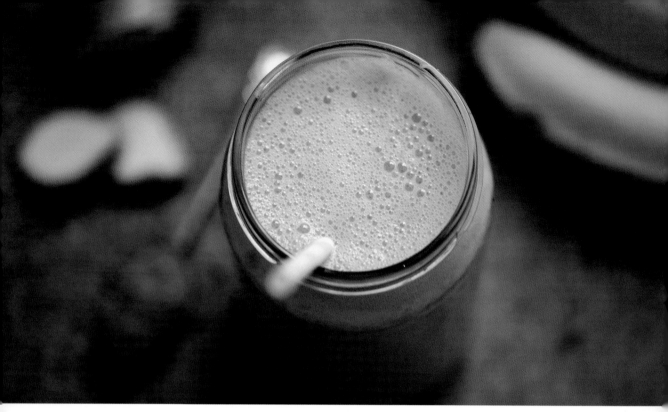

Turmeric Smoothie

Smoothies are a great way to get nutrients into your body for easier digestion. Turmeric, an anti-inflammatory spice, gives this creamy drink a golden glow. I've included a few substitutes for coconut milk, but the turmeric and coconut milk pair well together.

Makes 2 servings

1 cup Coconut Milk (page 15) or other SCD-legal coconut milk

2 bananas

2 teaspoons ground turmeric

½ teaspoon ground ginger

1 tablespoon honey

6 to 8 ice cubes

Place all the ingredients in a blender or food processor and blend until smooth.

Nutrition per serving: *176 calories, 3 g fat, 40 g carbohydrate, 4 g fiber, 2 g protein*

Tips

◆ You can substitute the coconut milk with dairy or dairy-free yogurt, Almond Milk (page 13), or Cashew Milk (page 16).

Salads and Soups

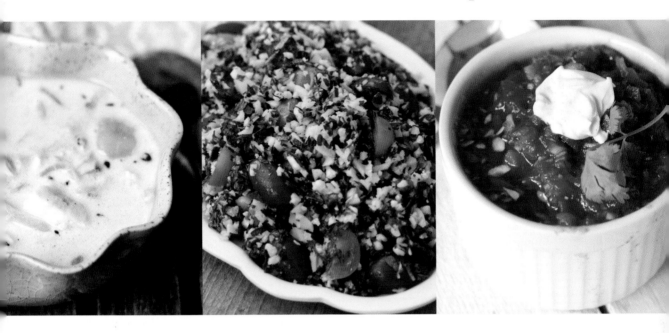

Soups are classic comfort food, and they're easy to digest. Besides the recipes in this chapter, you can make soups from the chicken, beef, and vegetable broths in the Basic Recipes chapter (page 10).

When it comes to salads, if you're not able to eat raw veggies and fruits, you can get creative by cooking your salads or letting them marinate in a dressing for a day to soften them up.

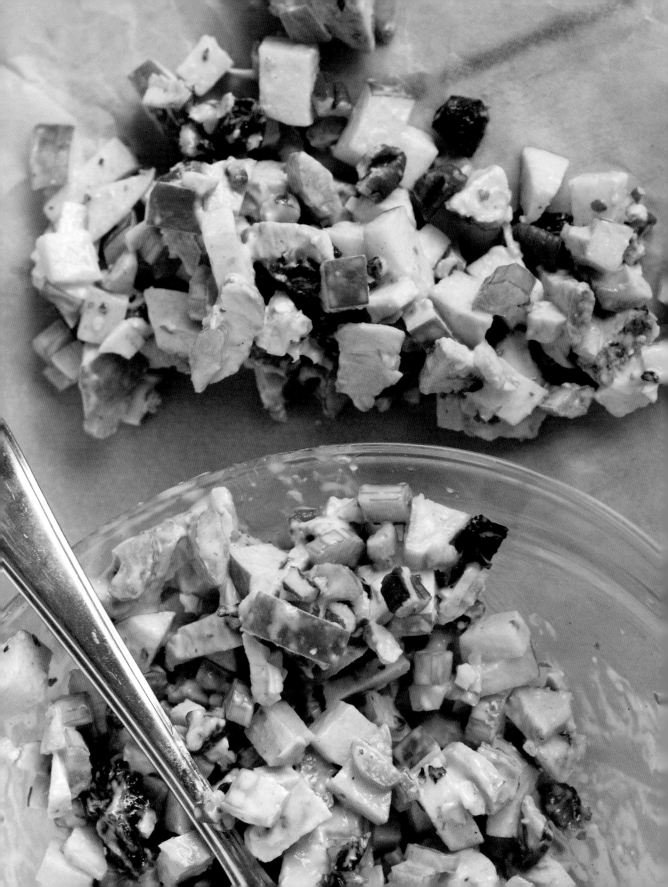

Cherry Chicken Salad

This creamy chopped salad is on the sweet side, and meant to be served cold, but it can be a bit less sweet if you choose a tart apple and tart cherries. If you're not eating raw fruits and veggies, steam the apples and celery for 5 minutes or so, or until tender. Then add them to the rest of the ingredients. You can soak the pecans as well, if you wish (see page 11).

Makes 4 (1-cup) servings

1 cup dried or pitted fresh cherries, finely chopped

2 cups chopped roasted chicken (or other cooked chicken)

½ cup finely chopped apples (peel or no peel, your choice)

½ cup finely chopped celery

¼ cup chopped raw or roasted pecans

2 tablespoons Mayonnaise (page 36)

1. If you're using dried cherries, soak them in a bowl of hot water (about the temperature of hot tap water) for about 10 minutes. Drain.

2. Combine all the ingredients in a bowl and stir to blend well.

3. Serve, or cover and store in the refrigerator for up to a few days.

> **Nutrition per serving:** *256 calories, 10 g fat, 36 g carbohydrate, 2 g fiber, 6 g protein*

Creamy Coleslaw

While I know that cabbage can be a bit hard on the digestive system, when you let coleslaw marinate for a few hours, or overnight, it loses that problematic crunch and firmness. This coleslaw works well as a side dish, as a topping for Fish Tacos (page 174) or grilled food, or on sandwiches. And even if you're feeling fine and are symptom free, letting the cabbage marinate in the dressing for a few hours makes it just that much better.

Makes 4 (1-cup) servings

½ medium green cabbage

½ medium red cabbage

½ cup mayonnaise

2 tablespoons vinegar (apple cider or white wine vinegar is good)

2 tablespoons Dijon mustard (or other mustard)

2 tablespoons honey

1. Using a food processor, thinly slice, dice, or shred the cabbage. Transfer the cut-up cabbage to a large mixing bowl.

2. Add all the remaining ingredients to the bowl and mix until well blended, adjusting the flavors to your liking. Cover and refrigerate the coleslaw for up to a week.

> **Nutrition per serving:** *301 calories, 23 g fat, 32 g carbohydrate, 6 g fiber, 4 g protein*

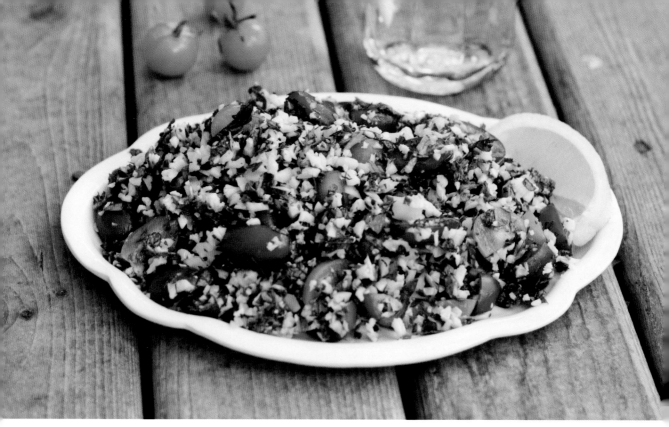

Tabbouleh

This classic Middle Eastern dish uses roasted cauliflower to bring rich flavor and texture similar to that of traditional tabbouleh made with bulgur or couscous. It's meant to be a parsley salad, but I tend to add more of all the other good stuff. If you want a more authentic salad, add another cup or so of fresh chopped parsley. If you're not eating raw veggies, you can give the veggies and herbs a quick stir-fry to soften them up before adding them to this salad.

Makes 4 (1-cup) servings

1 large cauliflower head (or 2 small heads), diced into small chunks

1 tablespoon ghee (page 23), high-heat oil, or coconut oil

¼ teaspoon sea salt, plus more as needed

2 cups finely chopped fresh parsley

1 cup finely chopped fresh mint

2 cups diced tomatoes (small pieces)

3 green onions, bottoms removed, thinly diced

1 tablespoon fresh lemon juice, plus more as needed

1 tablespoon olive oil

1. Preheat your oven to 400°F/200°C.

2. In a bowl, blend the cauliflower, ghee or oil, and salt together until the cauliflower is well coated.

3. Spread the cauliflower onto the baking sheet and roast for 20 minutes.

4. Let cool for a few minutes, then place in the bowl of a food processor and process into grain-size pieces.

5. Transfer the cauliflower to a bowl and add the parsley, mint, tomatoes, green onions, 1 tablespoon lemon juice, and the olive oil. Blend well, adjusting the seasoning with more salt and/or lemon juice, as desired.

6. Serve either chilled or at room temperature.

Nutrition per serving: *136 calories, 7 g fat, 15 g carbohydrate, 5 g fiber, 5 g protein*

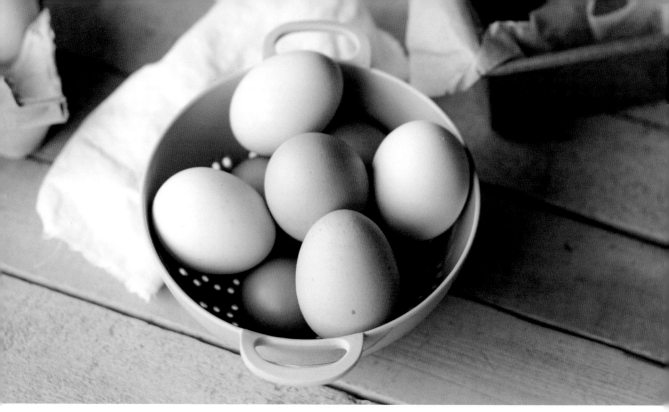

Scrambled Egg Salad

If you're craving egg salad but don't have time to hard-boil the eggs, try this quick and easy scrambled version.

Makes 2 servings

4 eggs, scrambled and chopped

2 tablespoons Mayonnaise (page 36), Crème Fraîche (page 24), or SCD Yogurt (page 20), plus more if needed

1 teaspoon honey (optional)

½ celery stalk, diced into small pieces

a few dill or other pickle slices, diced

salt and pepper, to taste

Place all the ingredients in a bowl and blend thoroughly. Add more mayonnaise as needed.

Nutrition per serving: *244 calories, 5 g fat, 4 g carbohydrate, 0 g fiber, 13 g protein*

Curried Egg Salad

This egg salad is a meal in itself, depending on what you add to the medley. Spread it on an Almond Saltine Cracker (page 48) or it on to some Simple Sandwich Bread (page 92). The dressing can be used with other salads, too. I like to add it to chopped-up leftover chicken and then blend in leftover fruits and vegetables. You can change this as you wish, so I've just listed a few suggestions. If you're still having symptoms, you'll want to add cooked rather than raw fruits and vegetables.

This dressing used is a very quick one that I make when I don't have mayonnaise on hand, but you could swap in mayonnaise if you don't have yogurt, or try the Curry Dressing on page 85 for a full-on version of my favorite dressing for this salad.

Makes 4 servings

SALAD

5 eggs

1 cup diced grapes (raisins or currants work, too; soak them in hot tap water for a few minutes to soften them), diced

¼ cup finely diced green onions or chives

½ cup finely chopped apples (peeled or not, your choice)

¼ cup soaked nuts (pistachios, pecans, almonds, or walnuts work well; see page 11 for soaking directions)

salt and pepper, to taste

DRESSING

½ cup SCD Yogurt (page 20)

1 teaspoon honey

½ teaspoon curry powder

1. Bring a large saucepan of water to a boil. Use a spoon to gently lower the eggs into the boiling water; they should be completely covered with water. Boil for 15 minutes and then immediately cool in ice water for 10 minutes.

2. Prepare the dressing by combining the yogurt, honey, curry powder, salt, and pepper in a small bowl, blending well with a fork or whisk.

3. Gently crack the sides of the eggs and peel off the shells. Chop the eggs into very small pieces.

4. In a bowl, combine the dressing with the chopped eggs and all the other ingredients, gently stirring with a spoon. Serve, or cover and store in the refrigerator for up to about a week.

> **Nutrition per serving:** *181 calories, 11 g fat, 12 g carbohydrate, 2 g fiber, 10 g protein*

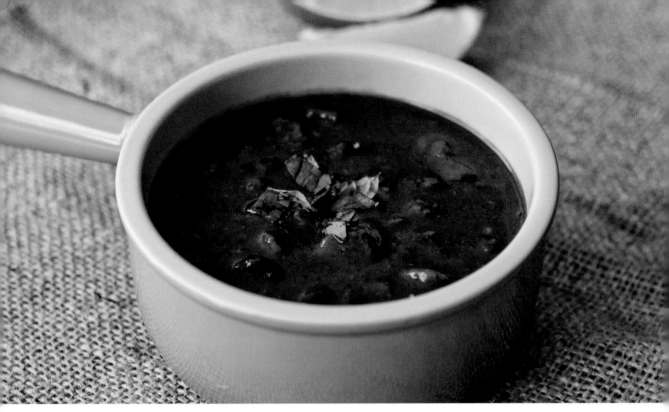

Black Bean Soup

Makes 6 servings

For a delicious meal, pair this soup with crème fraîche (page 24), yogurt, or Sour Cashew Cream (page 18); diced avocado; and a wedge of lime.

3 tablespoons olive oil (or other cooking oil)

1 large yellow onion, finely chopped

3 large carrots, peeled and cut into coins

1 large celery stalk, finely chopped

½ teaspoon salt

4 medium garlic cloves, minced

1 tablespoon ground cumin

1 teaspoon chili powder

4 cups Vegetable Broth (page 31, Chicken Broth (page 28), or water

1 tablespoon honey

2 cups black beans that have been rinsed and soaked in 4 quarts of water overnight, then washed and drained

1 red bell pepper, diced into small pieces

a few tablespoons lime juice, to taste

sea salt, to taste

1. Place the olive oil in a large saucepan (at least 6-quart size) over medium heat.

2. Place the carrots, onion, celery, and salt in the saucepan and cook for about 5 minutes, stirring occasionally, until the onion begins to turn translucent.

3. Add the garlic, cumin, and chili powder. Blend well and cook for a few minutes.

4. Add the broth, honey, and beans and stir to blend well. Bring to a boil and then reduce the heat, loosely cover, and simmer for about 1½ to 2 hours, or until beans are tender. Add the red bell pepper about 30 minutes before the soup is finished cooking.

5. Ladle out about half the soup into a blender container. Puree until smooth and then stir back into the soup in the saucepan.

6. Add lime juice and sea salt to taste and serve with your favorite toppings. The soup can be refrigerated for a few days or frozen for use later.

Nutrition per serving: *234 calories, 10 g fat, 31 g carbohydrate, 8 g fiber, 8 g protein*

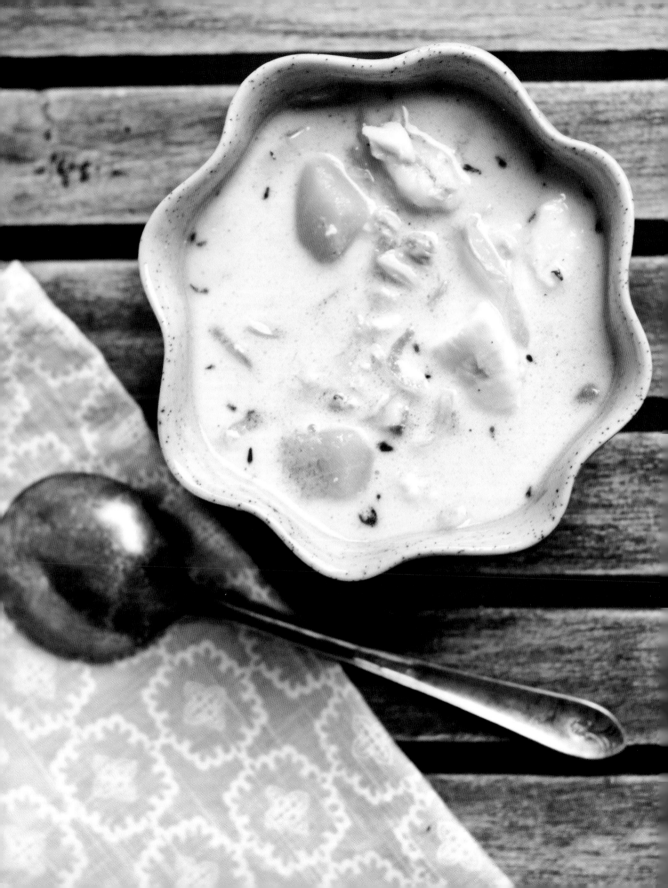

Seafood Chowder

When you're in the mood for a simple, wholesome serving of seafood chowder, this recipe will give you just that. Seafood chowder serves up a bowl full of easily digested vegetables, broth, and protein for healing and fortification.

This seafood chowder can easily be made dairy-free and you can use any seafood you have on hand in your freezer, or if you're lucky, fresh seafood. It seems to taste best on a blustery rainy day, with images of rough seas and storms in the background.

Makes 4 servings

1 tablespoon ghee (page 23), butter, or cooking oil

1 large yellow onion, chopped (about 2 cups)

1 cup peeled and diced winter squash (such as butternut or acorn) cut into bite-size pieces

2 cups clam juice (or fish stock)

1 tablespoon fresh thyme (or 1 teaspoon dried thyme)

1 teaspoon salt, plus more as needed

about 2 pounds raw seafood (such as shrimp, clams, cod, halibut), cut into bite-size pieces

1 cup Crème Fraîche (page 24), SCD Yogurt (page 20), or dairy-free milk

pepper, to taste

1. Heat the ghee, butter, or oil in a large saucepan over medium heat. Add the onion to the saucepan and heat for about 5 minutes, or until it starts to turn translucent.

2. Add the squash, clam juice or fish stock, thyme, and 1 teaspoon salt and bring to a low boil. Cook for about 10 minutes, or until the squash is somewhat tender.

3. Add the seafood and cook for another 5 minutes, or until all the seafood is cooked. Remove from the heat and let cool for a few minutes.

4. Stir the crème fraîche into the chowder and blend well. Season to taste with salt and pepper. Serve immediately, store in the refrigerator for up to several days, or freeze for up to a few weeks.

> **Nutrition per serving:** *257 calories, 6 g fat, 23 g carbohydrate, 3 g fiber, 29 g protein*

Tips

◆ If you don't have fish stock or fresh clam juice, you can use Vegetable Broth (page 31) or water.

Tomato Cheddar Basil Soup

Makes 4 servings

Cheese and tomato go well together in so many recipes, the first of which that comes to mind is pizza. But this is a close second in flavor, and you can up the ante by pairing it with Grilled Cheese Croutons (page 44) and garnishing with fresh basil.

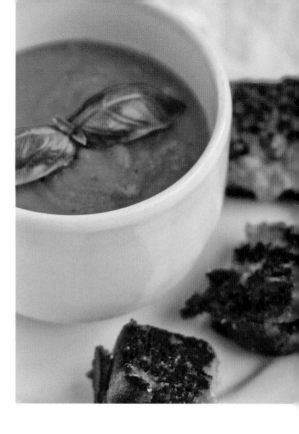

1 tablespoon ghee (page 23) or cooking oil

1 small yellow onion, chopped

1 garlic clove, chopped

3½ cups Tomato Sauce (page 35)

1 cup Vegetable Broth (page 31) or water

1 teaspoon dried oregano

about 6 fresh basil leaves, chopped (or about 1 teaspoon dried basil)

¼ teaspoon salt, plus more as needed

1 teaspoon honey

½ cup SCD Yogurt (page 20), dairy-free milk, or Sour Cashew Cream (page 18)

½ cup grated cheddar or other aged cheese, plus more for serving

salt and pepper, to taste

1. Warm the ghee or oil in a large saucepan over medium heat. Add the onion and cook for 5 minutes. Add the chopped garlic and cook for a few more minutes.

2. Add the tomato sauce, vegetable broth, oregano, basil, ¼ teaspoon salt, and honey to the saucepan and stir to blend well. Bring to a boil, reduce the heat, and then simmer, covered, for about 10 minutes.

3. Let cool for few minutes and then add the yogurt and cheese. Puree the soup using a blender, food processor, or immersion blender. Season with salt and pepper to taste.

4. Garnish individual servings with additional shredded cheese.

5. Store in the refrigerator for up to a few days, or freeze for a month or so.

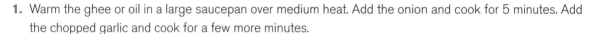

Nutrition per serving: *185 calories, 9 g fat, 20 g carbohydrate, 3 g fiber, 8 g protein*

French Onion Soup

Any recipe with caramelized onions is probably one that I'll love, including this classic soup. French onion soup requires you to set aside a couple of hours to make it, but I think it's well worth the time it takes.

I've simplified this recipe a bit, mostly by toasting the bread and cheese separately from the bowl of soup. If you prefer, you can ladle soup into an oven-safe bowl, top it with toasted bread and grated cheese, and bake it in your oven for about 10 minutes at 350°F/175°C.

Makes 4 servings

3 large red or yellow onions (about 1 pound), thinly sliced

2 tablespoons olive oil, ghee (page 23), or butter (or some combination)

drizzle of honey

½ teaspoon salt, plus more as needed

1 garlic clove, minced

6 cups broth (beef, chicken, or vegetable)

¼ cup dry white wine (optional)

pepper, to taste

4 slices Simple Sandwich Bread (page 92)

½ cup grated Gruyère or other Swiss cheese

1. Place the onions and oil, ghee, or butter in a large saucepan or Dutch oven over low heat. Cover and cook for 15 minutes.

2. Raise the heat to medium-low, add the honey and ½ teaspoon salt, and stir to dissolve. With the cover off, cook the onions for 30 to 40 minutes more, or until they are caramelized (they'll turn brown, gooey, and sweet). Stir occasionally.

3. Add the garlic and cook for 1 minute.

4. Add the broth and wine, if using, and stir to blend. Add salt and pepper to taste, cover, and simmer for 30 minutes, partially covered to allow some moisture to escape.

5. Cover the bread with the grated cheese and toast in the oven on broil or a high heat setting for about 5 minutes, or until the cheese is bubbling and turning darker and the edges of the bread are crisp.

6. To serve, fill four bowls with the onion soup and place a piece of cheese bread on top of each.

Nutrition per serving: *264 calories, 13 g fat, 23 g carbohydrate, 2 g fiber, 9 g protein*

Tips
◆ To make this vegetarian, use Vegetable Broth (page 31) and add 2 to 3 tablespoons of Mock Soy Sauce (page 89).

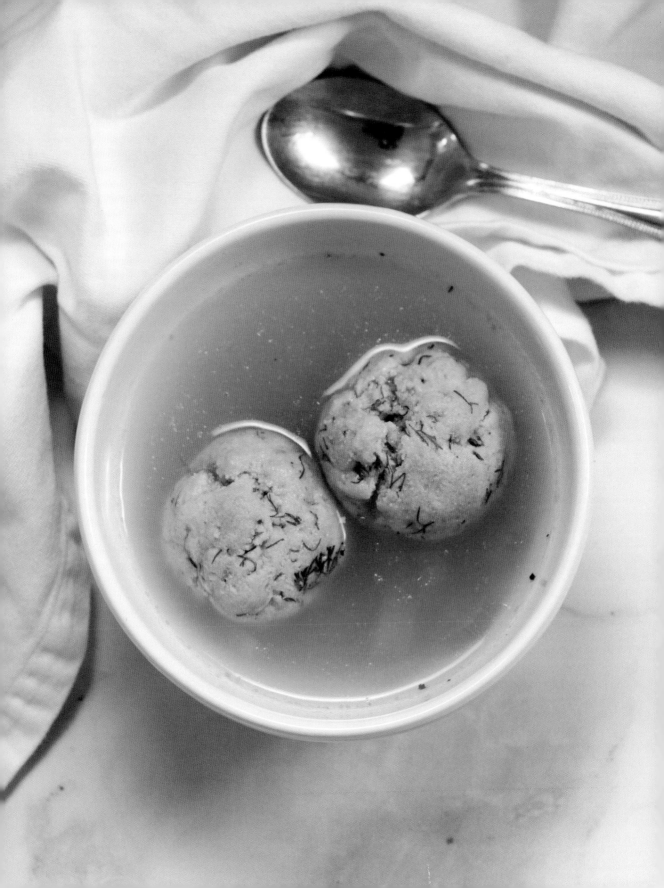

Matzo Ball Soup (Coconut Flour)

Chicken soup, also known as Jewish penicillin, is even better with the addition of 1 or 2 matzo balls. This nut-free matzo ball soup recipe can be made dairy-free by replacing the butter with coconut oil or other dairy-free fat. For the herbs, I like using dill, thyme, or sage, and a pinch of black pepper.

Makes 8 dumplings

4 eggs

¼ cup unsalted butter, melted

¼ teaspoon salt

¼ teaspoon baking soda

¼ cup coconut flour

2 teaspoons dried herbs or 2 tablespoons fresh chopped herbs

8 cups Chicken Broth (page 28)

1. Preheat the oven to 350°F/175°C.

2. Line a baking sheet with parchment paper or a nonstick baking mat.

3. In a medium bowl, add all the ingredients, except the chicken broth. Mix well with a spoon.

4. Scoop 1 to 2 tablespoons batter into a ball, roll in your hands, and place on the baking sheet. Repeat for the remaining batter.

5. Bake for 12 to 15 minutes or until the balls are firm enough to hold their shape.

6. Serve with very warm chicken broth.

Nutrition per dumpling: *157 calories, 3 g carbohydrate, 9 g fat, 9 g protein, 2 g fiber*

Tips

♦ If you'd prefer, you can drop the matzo balls into the soup to cook because they are a bit more delicate when firming them up in the soup. If you do this, place the matzo balls in the freezer for at least 10 minutes to get them firm. When ready to cook, gently lower the balls into the simmering broth with a spoon.

♦ For a lighter, less dense dough, add another 2 eggs to the recipe for a total of 6 eggs and use a spoon to drop the batter onto the baking sheet.

Matzo Ball Soup (Almond Flour)

I love this recipe because it's so simple. Use any herbs or spices you prefer (I tend to use dried dill and basil), or just add some black pepper.

Makes 10 dumplings

2 cups almond flour

1 teaspoon salt

2 eggs

1 teaspoon dried herbs

8 cups Chicken Broth (page 28)

1. Preheat the oven to 350°F/175°C.

2. Line a baking sheet with parchment paper or a nonstick baking mat.

3. Add all the ingredients except the broth to a medium bowl and mix well with a spoon.

4. Scoop 1 to 2 tablespoons of batter into a ball, roll in your hands, and place on the baking sheet. Repeat for the remaining batter.

5. Bake for 12 to 15 minutes or until the balls are firm enough to hold their shape.

6. Serve with very warm chicken broth.

Nutrition per dumpling: *157 calories, 3 g carbohydrate, 9 g fat, 9 g protein, 2 g fiber*

Tips

◆ If you'd prefer, you can drop the matzo balls into the soup to cook because they are a bit more delicate when firming them up in the soup. If you do this, place the matzo balls in the freezer for at least 10 minutes to get them firm. When they are ready to cook, gently lower the balls into the simmering broth with a spoon.

◆ For a lighter, less dense dough, add another 2 eggs to the recipe for a total of 4 eggs, and use a spoon to drop the batter onto the baking sheet.

Gazpacho

This chilled tomato-based soup is a wonderful way to cool down during the summer. The method I've given here is a classic one, but the soup can also be blended into more of a smoothie consistency. Ideally, you'll want to chill this soup for at least an hour before serving, or overnight. It gets better when it marinates for a while. When you're ready to serve your gazpacho you can add diced avocado, diced onion, and Crème Fraîche (page 24) to enhance it. It makes a fine accompaniment to grilled chicken, shrimp, or steak.

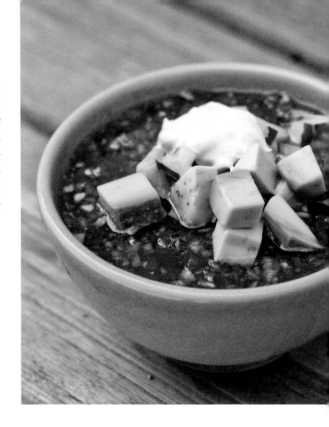

Makes 4 servings

> 1 large cucumber, peeled and cut into large pieces
>
> 1 large red bell pepper, cut into large pieces
>
> 4 plum tomatoes, cut into large pieces
>
> 1 medium red onion, cut into large pieces
>
> 2 garlic cloves
>
> 1 cup tomato juice (or ½ cup tomato puree and ½ cup water)
>
> 2 tablespoons red or white wine vinegar
>
> 2 tablespoons olive oil
>
> 1 teaspoon sea salt
>
> dash of red Tabasco sauce (no additives or preservatives), or pinch of cayenne pepper (optional)

1. In a food processor, separately pulse the following into finely ground pieces: cucumber, tomatoes, and red bell pepper. Place in a large mixing bowl.

2. Pulse the onion and garlic together into finely ground pieces and add to the tomato mixture.

3. Stir the remaining ingredients into the tomato mixture, blending well. Cover and refrigerate to serve chilled.

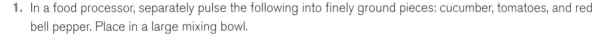

Nutrition per serving: *117 calories, 7 g fat, 11 g carbohydrate, 3 g fiber, 3 g protein*

Italian Wedding Soup

There are many variations on this soup, but essentially they all come down to broth with greens, veggies, and meatballs. This is a very nurturing soup that can serve as a hearty meal on its own. The meatballs are the Fennel Pesto Meatballs on page 162 served with tomato sauce; when I'm making those, I double the recipe and use half for this soup. You can refrigerate or freeze half of this soup for another time.

Makes 6 servings

2 tablespoons ghee (page 23) or cooking oil

1 small yellow onion, finely diced

1 medium carrot, peeled and finely chopped

1 stalk celery, finely chopped

2 medium garlic cloves, finely minced

8 cups chicken or vegetable broth

1 cup chopped spinach, kale, or other greens (cut in bite-size pieces)

½ teaspoon dried thyme (or ½ tablespoon of fresh)

½ teaspoon dried oregano (or ½ tablespoon of fresh)

¼ teaspoon salt, plus more as needed

1 recipe Fennel Pesto Meatballs (page 162)

pepper, to taste

⅓ cup grated Parmesan cheese, for serving (optional)

Garlic Toasts (page 120) or Parmesan Crackers (page 46), for serving (optional)

1. Add the ghee or oil to the pan along with the onion, carrot, celery, and garlic. Cook for a few minutes, stirring occasionally.

2. Stir in the broth, chopped greens, thyme, oregano, and salt, blending well. Spoon the meatballs into the broth. Simmer for 30 minutes, or until the vegetables are tender. Adjust the seasoning with salt and pepper to taste.

3. Place the soup in a serving bowl and top with shredded Parmesan and croutons, if you wish, or offer the toasts. This soup can be refrigerated for a few days, covered, or kept in the freezer for a few months.

Nutrition per serving: *330 calories, 27 g fat, 8 g carbohydrate, 1 g fiber, 18 g protein*

Mushroom Soup (Dairy-Free)

This soup has the earthy flavor of mushrooms and the creamy consistency of dairy-free cashew cream. Most mushrooms in the store are the same variety (cremini, white, Portobello). The difference between them is their age: The younger mushrooms are lighter in color. I use cremini for this recipe.

Makes 4 servings

3 tablespoons olive oil

1 pound cremini mushrooms, sliced or chopped

2 shallots, chopped

2 cloves garlic, chopped

3 cups Vegetable Broth (page 31) or water

1 ½ teaspoons salt or to taste

½ teaspoon dried thyme or tarragon

1 cup Simple Cashew Cream (page 19)

pepper, to taste

1. Place a large stockpot on medium heat and add olive oil, mushrooms, shallots, and garlic.

2. Sauté the mushrooms for 10 minutes or until the moisture from the mushrooms is mostly cooked off.

3. Add the vegetable broth, salt, and thyme. Simmer for 5 minutes, turn the heat off, and add the cashew cream.

4. Let the soup cool for a few minutes before blending it in small batches. You can blend part of it and leave some mushroom pieces, or blend all of it until smooth.

5. Serve hot. Store leftovers in the refrigerator for a few days or freeze for a few months.

> **Nutrition per serving:** *131 calories, 12 g fat, 8 g carbohydrate, 1 g fiber, 5 g protein*

Tips

♦ To make this nut-free, substitute the Simple Cashew Cream with steamed cauliflower (steam half a head until tender, cool, then pulse in a blender or food processor until creamy).

♦ If you'd like to add some very dry white cooking wine, which is SCD legal, use about 2 tablespoons in step 2.

Broccoli Cheddar Soup

The cheddar cheese may be the star in this dish, but the addition of carrots adds a thicker consistency and sweetness, which plays off the salty cheddar cheese.

Makes 4 servings

1 tablespoon olive oil

1 large yellow onion, diced

¾ teaspoon salt, divided

2 carrots, peeled, trimmed, and sliced into coins

10 ounces broccoli florets (fresh or frozen)

2 to 3 cups water or Vegetable Broth (page 31)

6 ounces (about 2 cups) cheddar cheese, shredded

1. Warm a saucepan on medium-low heat and then add the olive oil.

2. Sauté the onion and ¼ teaspoon salt until the onions begin to brown, about 8 minutes.

3. Add the carrots and broccoli plus enough water to bring the vegetables to a boil.

4. Cover the saucepan, reduce to low, and simmer for about 12 minutes, or until the broccoli and carrots are tender.

5. Turn off the heat, take the cover off, and add the cheese and remaining ½ teaspoon salt. Stir until the cheese has melted. Add more water if you prefer a thinner consistency.

6. Cool for a bit and then blend the soup in batches until smooth or at the consistency you prefer.

7. Serve warm. Store in the refrigerator for a few days or freeze for a few months.

Nutrition per serving: *249 calories, 19 g fat, 7 g carbohydrate, 3 g fiber, 11 g protein*

Tips

♦ I recommend a mild, aged white cheddar rather than a very sharp one, which can create a slightly bitter cheese taste in the soup.

Sauces, Jams, and Dips

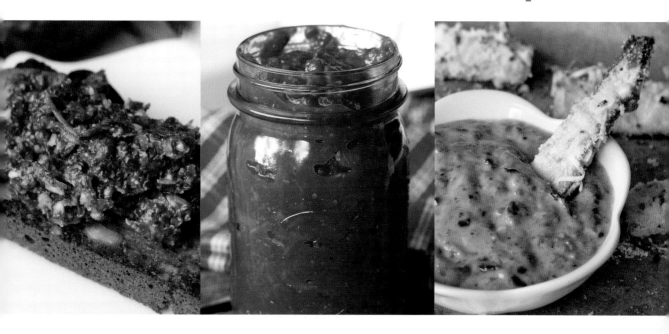

Here are some of my favorite sauces, with a range of textures and flavors to accompany a variety of foods. You'll want to make extra of some of these classic sauces—such as the homemade ketchup and the marinara sauce—and freeze them so you'll have them on hand to use later.

Classic Marinara Sauce

This vitamin-rich tomato sauce can be used for all sorts of recipes that call for tomato sauce. I use cans of crushed tomatoes, but if Roma (plum) tomatoes are in season, find a way to buy a few pounds and run them through a food mill, and you'll end up with the most fantastic marinara sauce. Roma tomatoes, in season, are among the sweetest and most flavorful tomatoes around. Try to buy organic tomatoes or sauce, if possible; since tomato skins are thin, it's likely the insides will absorb any toxins or pesticides. The grated carrots are my favorite ingredient in this recipe. They give a vitamin boost and sweeten the sauce.

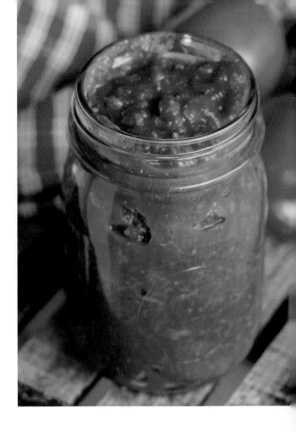

Makes 12 cups

¼ cup olive oil

1 small onion, finely diced (about 1 cup)

4 garlic cloves, minced

7 cups Tomato Sauce (page 35)

½ cup finely grated peeled carrots (about 2 small carrots)

1 teaspoon dried basil (or a few fresh leaves, chopped)

¼ teaspoon sea salt, plus more as needed

1 teaspoon dried oregano

pinch of red pepper flakes (optional, for a little kick)

pepper, to taste

1. Place the olive oil, onion, and garlic in a large saucepan and heat over low to medium heat. Cook until the onions begin to soften, or for about 5 minutes.

2. Add the tomatoes, carrots, basil, salt, oregano, and red pepper flakes, if using, and stir to blend well.

3. Bring the sauce to a boil and then reduce to a steady simmer and cover the saucepan. Simmer for at least 30 minutes, stirring occasionally. Season to taste with salt and pepper.

4. Cover and store the sauce in the refrigerator; it will keep for about a week. You can also freeze this sauce for up to 6 months, or can it for a year.

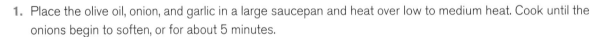

Nutrition per cup: *83 calories, 5 g fat, 9 g carbohydrate, 2 g fiber, 2 g protein*

Honey Mustard Dressing and Dip

This somewhat thick dressing also makes a great dip for veggies and Chicken Tenders (page 150). The recipe calls for mayonnaise, but you can substitute Sour Cashew Cream (page 18) or olive oil if you wish.

I like this dressing on the sweet side, so I use close to 2 tablespoons of honey. If you're not sure, start with 1 tablespoon, taste, and then add more if desired. This recipe can easily be doubled.

Makes 8 tablespoons

> ¼ cup Mayonnaise (page 36)
>
> 2 tablespoons stoneground mustard (or other prepared mustard)
>
> 1 ½ tablespoons honey, or to taste

Combine all the ingredients in a bowl and whisk or stir until completely blended. Store in the refrigerator in a sealed container for a few weeks.

***

Nutrition per tablespoon: *57 calories, 5 g fat, 3 g carbohydrate, 1 g fiber, 1 g protein*

***

Reduced Toxic Load

Every day you are breathing, drinking, and absorbing all kinds of chemicals. Some are naturally occurring while others aren't, and you probably don't want the latter near you or inside you. While they may be present only in small amounts, over time these harmful chemicals can accumulate in your body and create a toxic load that affects how you feel and live. Here are a few ways to lower your toxic load: drink filtered water; use green cleaning products, soaps, shampoos, and other personal care products (see ewg.org/skindeep); wear and use natural fabrics and other products with low to no toxicity; eat organic food when possible; avoid antibiotics, pesticides, and industrially produced food.

Simple Ketchup

There are a lot of good ketchup recipes, but this one is quite simple, which is why I like it. You can make tomato paste by simmering tomato juice for an hour or so, or until it has the consistency of tomato paste—just keep the top off the saucepan. In a pinch you can use tomato sauce in this recipe and let it simmer longer to condense it to the thickness you desire.

Makes 16 tablespoons

1 cup (8 ounces) Tomato Paste (page 35)

¼ teaspoon apple cider vinegar

1 teaspoon honey (optional for a sweeter ketchup)

water, if needed

1. Place all the ingredients in a saucepan over a low to medium heat and simmer for 10 minutes or so, stirring occasionally to blend. Add a little water if the ketchup becomes thicker than you want.

2. Let cool to room temperature, cover, and refrigerate. This ketchup will keep for about a week or so in the refrigerator, and you can freeze some for later use.

> **Nutrition per tablespoon:** *16 calories, 0 g fat, 3 g carbohydrate, 1 g fiber, 1 g protein*

Avoid Additives and Processed Food

When you read the label of a packaged or canned food, if there are ingredients you don't recognize or you're unsure if they're OK to eat while following SCD, then steer clear of these foods. Finding fresh, unpackaged, and minimally processed foods is your goal. Eating seasonal and organic food is a bonus, because you're reducing your toxic load and getting the maximum nutrients from the food.

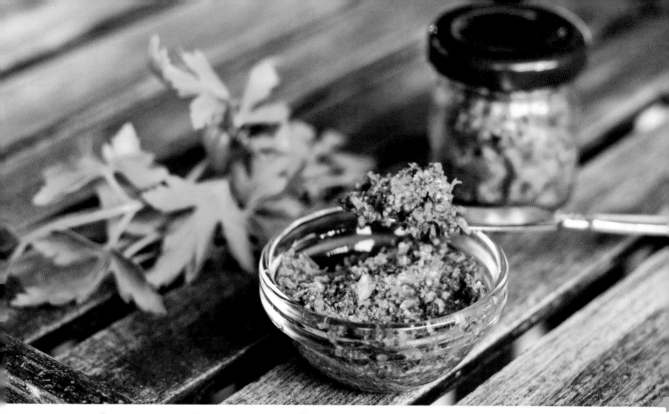

Parsley and Spinach Pesto

The real trick to making good pesto is to have a food processor. Because I like to make pesto at a moment's notice, I keep these basic ingredients on hand: Parmesan cheese, fresh lemon, and olive oil. Then I take whatever greens I happen to have, and green onions if I have them, and it all goes together in the food processor. My favorite fresh greens for making pesto are arugula, spinach, parsley, basil, and mixed baby greens. The parsley in the following recipe helps prevent the pesto from turning brownish green. Keep this pesto around for a meal at any time—green eggs, green cauliflower rice, fish or chicken marinade, or simply a spread for pizza crust or toast. If you don't eat Parmesan or other hard aged cheese, you can substitute pine nuts (which are actually seeds) and salt. I use about ¼ cup pine nuts and ⅛ teaspoon sea salt when I don't have Parmesan on hand.

Makes 4 (¼-cup) servings

4 ounces (or so) fresh parsley

4 ounces (or so) fresh spinach

2 green onions, cut into segments

¼ cup olive oil (or more if needed)

2 garlic cloves

¼ cup grated or shredded Parmesan cheese

¼ teaspoon salt

1. Whirl the parsley and spinach in a food processor until finely chopped.

2. Add all the remaining ingredients and process until finely ground and well blended. Store in the refrigerator, sealed, for up to a week or so, or freeze for up to a few months.

Nutrition per serving: *250 calories, 21 g fat, 6 g carbohydrate, 2 g fiber, 11 g protein*

Basil Walnut Pesto (Dairy-Free)

Slight confession here: I often eat pesto without much else. All the green herbs, healthy fats, and lemon juice hit the spot for me. This is my favorite way to make pesto because it's so simple, and completely plant-based. The walnuts create a great consistency and offer a good dose of healthy fat.

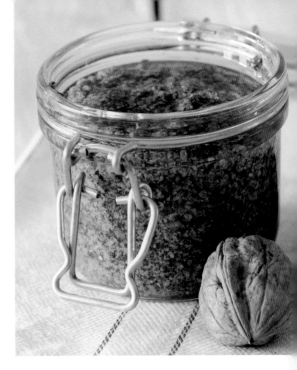

Makes 4 (¼-cup) servings

4 ounces basil leaves

½ cup chopped walnuts

2 tablespoons lemon juice

1 tablespoon olive oil

⅛ teaspoon salt

1 clove garlic (optional)

Add all the ingredients to a food processor or high-speed blender and blend well. Store covered in the refrigerator for a week or so.

Nutrition per serving: *139 calories, 13 g fat, 4 g carbohydrate, 1 g fiber, 3 g protein*

Tips

- ♦ To prepare the basil, pinch the basil leaves off the stem with your fingers.
- ♦ To make this nut-free, substitute walnuts with pine nuts, which are considered seeds, or just leave out the nuts altogether and add more basil and olive oil.
- ♦ You can toast the walnuts for a deeper flavor.

Ranch Dressing

Here's a simple, creamy dressing or dip that can be used on salads, with chips and veggie strips, and with grilled meat strips. And what I love about this dressing is that while no buttermilk is necessary, it certainly tastes like it's in there. To make this dairy-free, replace the mayonnaise and yogurt with Sour Cashew Cream (page 18).

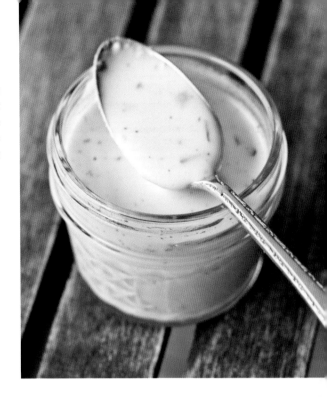

Makes 16 tablespoons

¼ cup mayonnaise

¼ cup SCD Yogurt (page 20)

2 teaspoons fresh lemon juice

¼ teaspoon garlic powder

¼ teaspoon onion powder

¼ teaspoon sea salt

1 tablespoon finely chopped fresh dill, Italian parsley, or chives (optional)

pepper, to taste

Combine all the ingredients in a bowl and blend well, using a fork or whisk. Cover and store in the refrigerator for up to a few weeks.

Nutrition per tablespoon: *49 calories, 3 g fat, 6 g carbohydrate, 1 g fiber, 1 g protein*

Ranch Dressing (Dairy-Free)

This is my favorite creamy, dairy-free dressing. It's so versatile: You can use it in sauces, marinades, as sour cream, as a dip, and more. The trick to preparing cashews for dairy-free recipes is to presoak them in water.

Makes 2 cups (32 tablespoons)

1 cup raw cashews

¾ cup water, plus more for soaking

½ teaspoon salt

2 to 3 tablespoons lemon juice

¼ teaspoon garlic powder

¼ teaspoon onion powder

1 tablespoon fresh dill leaves

1 tablespoon fresh parsley leaves

1. Soak the cashews in tap water for a few hours or hot water for 20 minutes. Remove and rinse the nuts.

2. Put the soaked cashews and ¾ cup water in a high-speed blender or food processor, and blend until creamy.

3. Add the salt, lemon juice, garlic powder, onion powder, dill, and parsley, and pulse to blend.

4. Use for salads, dips, and as a sauce. Store sealed in the refrigerator for a few weeks.

Nutrition per tablespoon: *21 calories, 2 g fat, 1 g carbohydrate, 0 g fiber, 1 g protein*

Tips

◆ This dressing is on the thick side, so you can easily thin it out with water while blending it, or stir in more water after.

Curry Dressing

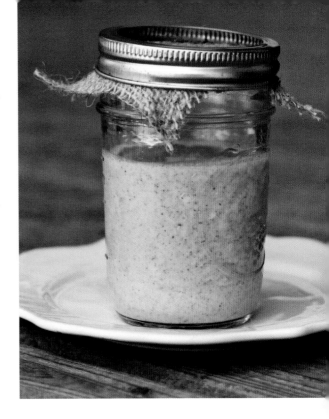

I love this dressing so much that I drink it—a bit. I sip it every now and then, and I lick the salad bowl to get every last drop of dressing after the salad morsels have been consumed. It seems to go with almost any fresh dish. Use it as a salad dressing, as a veggie and fruit dip, or as a super-tasty mayonnaise. It's especially good for chicken and egg salads.

If you're a bit sensitive to spicy seasonings, go a little easy on the curry powder. I tend to use a lot here, but you can still have great flavor using a teaspoon less.

Makes 16 (1-tablespoon) servings

⅓ cup Mayonnaise (page 36)

⅓ cup SCD Yogurt (page 20)

2 teaspoons honey

½ tablespoon lime juice (optional)

2 teaspoons curry powder

¼ teaspoon ground ginger

⅛ teaspoon sea salt

Combine all the ingredients in a bowl and blend well, using a fork or a whisk. Cover and store in the refrigerator for up to a few weeks.

Nutrition per serving: *49 calories, 3 g fat, 6 g carbohydrate, 1 g fiber, 1 g protein*

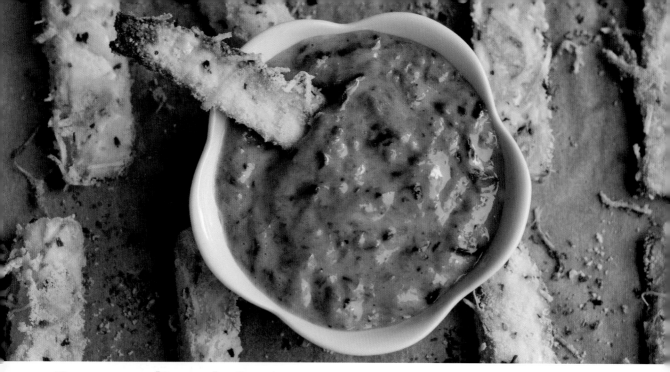

Caramelized Onion Dip

Caramelized anything sounds good to me, but especially caramelized onions. Use this dip for Zucchini Sticks (page 40), cut veggies, chicken strips, and other savory treats. It's also tasty as a spread on sandwiches.

Makes 8 (¼-cup) servings

1 large sweet onion (about 1 pound), diced

sea salt, as needed

1 tablespoon ghee (page 23), unsalted butter, or high-heat oil

2 tablespoons apple cider vinegar

2 tablespoons honey

1 tablespoon smooth mustard (Dijon works well)

1 cup Mayonnaise (page 36)

pepper, to taste

1. Place the onions, a pinch of salt, and the ghee, butter, or oil in a skillet over medium heat. Cook for about 15 minutes, stirring occasionally, until the onions are soft, translucent, and browned (caramelized).

2. Let cool and then combine the onions with the vinegar, honey, and mustard in a food processor or blender. Process until mostly smooth.

3. Transfer the onion mixture to a bowl and stir in the mayonnaise to blend well. Add salt and pepper to taste. Store sealed in the refrigerator for up to a few weeks.

> **Nutrition per serving:** *222 calories, 21 g fat, 7 g carbohydrate, 0 g fiber, 0 g protein*

Avocado Crema

Avocado crema isn't just for tacos and nachos, but it does a great job of serving those up. Try it on sandwiches, as a substitute for mayonnaise, and in dressings. This recipe can be made lactose-free by using crème fraîche or dairy-free by using Sour Cashew Cream. I kept this version mellow, but to spice it up, you can add a tablespoon of minced jalapeno (seeds removed for less kick) or a pinch of cayenne pepper.

This recipe makes 2 cups, but in my experience there's never enough, so I'd double this amount for a crowd.

Makes 8 (¼ cup) servings

1 ½ cups avocado pieces (about 2 avocados)

½ cup Crème Fraîche (page 24) or Sour Cashew Cream (page 18)

1 ½ tablespoons fresh lime juice

⅛ teaspoon salt, or to taste

Combine all the ingredients in a food processor, or blend them by hand using a potato smasher or fork, and process or blend until smooth. You can store the mixture in the refrigerator, covered, for about a week.

> **Nutrition per serving:** *91 calories, 9 g fat, 3 g carbohydrate, 2 g fiber, 1 g protein*

Always Make Extra

Leftovers are a great way to carry your meal planning over to the next day. Leftovers from dinner can be lunch for the next day. And don't restrict yourself to eating certain foods only at certain times of the day. Breakfast is okay for dinner, and vice versa.

Gravy

Here is one of my favorite gravy recipes using a few basic ingredients: pan drippings, cauliflower, stock, and shallots.

Makes 8 (½ cup) servings

2 tablespoons roasted chicken (or turkey) pan drippings

2 shallots, peeled and sliced

2 cups chopped raw cauliflower florets

2 cups Chicken Broth (page 28)

¼ teaspoon salt or to taste

1. Place a saucepan on medium-low heat.

2. Add the pan drippings, shallots, and cauliflower to the pan, and sauté for a few minutes or until the shallots begin to wilt.

3. Add the chicken broth and salt, and simmer covered until the cauliflower is tender, about 10 minutes.

4. Remove from the heat and cool for a few minutes.

5. Add the mixture to a blender or food processor in batches, blending until the gravy is creamy.

6. Add more broth or warm water if it's too thick.

7. Serve warm. Store in the refrigerator for a few days.

Nutrition per serving: *59 calories, 4 g fat, 3 g carbohydrate, 1 g fiber, 2 g protein*

Tips

♦ If you don't have pan drippings handy, use olive oil or butter.

♦ If you have leftover roasted chicken in the refrigerator, you can use the gelatin that settles to the bottom to add more flavor or as a substitute for pan drippings.

Mock Soy Sauce

If you're craving soy sauce, this mock version is a great substitute. Use it in any dish that calls for fish sauce, soy sauce, or tamari. It's also excellent in soups, stews, or salad dressings. I use it in fried cauliflower rice dishes, and in Asian-style sauces and dips.

Makes 3½ cups (2 tablespoons per serving)

¼ cup red wine vinegar

4 tablespoons honey

¼ teaspoon ginger, peeled and minced

2 cloves garlic, crushed

3 cups water

1 teaspoon salt

1. Combine all the ingredients in a saucepan and simmer over medium heat for 20 minutes, or until it's reduced by at least a half.

2. Store in the refrigerator for a few weeks.

> **Nutrition per serving:** *10 calories, 0 g fat, 3 g carbohydrate, 0 g fiber, 0 g protein*

Tartar Sauce

Here's a creamy, tart sauce that you can pair with fish, chicken, and vegetables as a dip or spread. It goes great with the Fish Sticks on page 176. Optionally, you can season this sauce with salt and pepper, and add a dash of hot sauce or the Mock Soy Sauce on page 89.

Makes 16 (1¼-tablespoon) servings

1 cup Mayonnaise (page 36)

¼ cup chopped dill pickles

1 teaspoon mustard

1 tablespoon fresh dill or tarragon (or a mix of both)

1 tablespoon fresh parsley

2 tablespoons capers, drained

1 tablespoon lemon juice

1. Add all the ingredients to a food processor or blender and pulse a few times to blend.

2. Store in the refrigerator for a week or so.

> **Nutrition per serving:** *91 calories, 10 g fat, 0 g carbohydrate, 0 g fiber, 0 g protein*

Strawberry Freezer Jam

This quick and easy strawberry jam recipe does away with the hassle of canning. Use fresh or frozen strawberries or really any berry or mixture of berries. It's great on a slice of toast, over yogurt, on pancakes, or over ice cream. You can also use it when baking.

Makes 16 (⅛-cup) servings

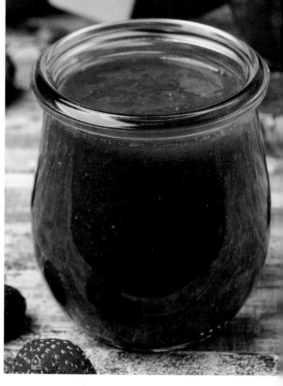

2 cups hulled strawberries

1 tablespoon lemon juice

1 cup honey

1. Place the strawberries in a food processor or blender and puree until mostly smooth. You can also mash them with a potato masher.

2. Combine the mashed strawberries, lemon juice, and honey in a saucepan and bring to a steady low boil.

3. Simmer for 30 minutes, or until the volume decreases by a third.

4. Cool to room temperature and place in a jar or container with a lid, leaving some space at the top for freezing expansion if you're freezing it. It keeps for about 2 weeks in the refrigerator or a few months in the freezer.

Nutrition per serving: *65 calories, 0 g fat, 18 g carbohydrate, 0 g fiber, 0 g protein*

Breads, Biscuits, and Crêpes

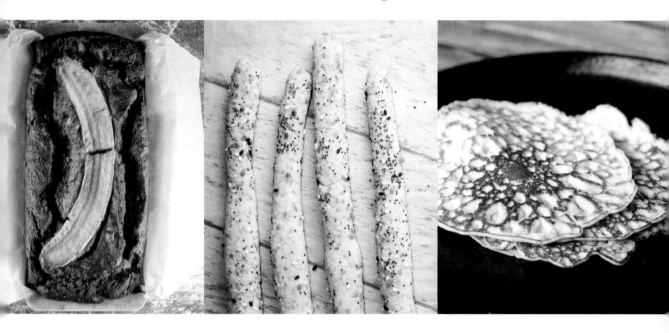

You'll find a lot of meal options in this chapter, many of them made with almond flour and/or coconut flour, or with nut butter. I prefer simple recipes, so my goal is that you'll find these easy to make and will stock up so that you always have something around for a quick meal or treat.

Simple Sandwich Bread

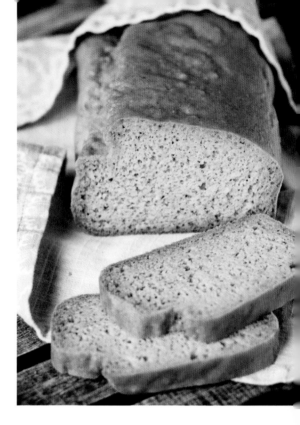

This is probably my favorite easy-to-bake bread. It can be used for sandwiches, rolls, and toast. It comes together easily and tastes delicious. What I also like about this bread is its overall texture, which to me is like sandwich bread that contains gluten. It stays together well, and it's a bit firm on the outside and softer on the inside. This is also a very flexible recipe, in that you can use just about any nut or seed butter. The flavor and color may change a bit, but the overall texture stays the same. If the nut butter is dark, like roasted almond butter, the bread will be on the darker side, while the opposite is true for lighter butters, such as cashew. Double the recipe to make more than one loaf at a time.

If you like French toast, create a loaf especially for French toast by adding an additional ½ tablespoon honey and 1 teaspoon ground cinnamon to the batter. Slice the bread, dip each slice in a beaten egg, and fry on both sides in a buttered frying pan.

Makes 10 slices

¾ cup smooth nut butter (I use almond or cashew)

4 eggs

1 tablespoon honey

¼ cup finely ground nut flour (I use blanched almond or cashew flour)

¼ teaspoon baking soda

1. Preheat your oven to 350°F/175°C.

2. In a bowl, use a spatula or mixer to blend together the nut butter, eggs, and honey until creamy.

3. Add the remaining dry ingredients to the batter and blend until creamy.

4. Pour the batter into a baking pan; I use a 3½ x 7½-inch loaf pan, but you can use a larger pan. Bake for 40 minutes, or until a toothpick inserted in the center of the loaf comes out clean.

5. Let cool and slice. Seal and store at room temperature for a few days, in the refrigerator for a few weeks, or in the freezer for a month or so.

Nutrition per slice: *147 calories, 11 g fat, 7 g carbohydrate, 2 g fiber, 6 g protein*

Sandwich Rounds

While you can use another of the breads in this book to make sandwich rolls, this is my favorite recipe for making flat rolls. It produces a sandwich round that tastes like a white roll and is easy to dress up. This isn't a high roll—it's more of a "round"— but I use these as rolls, and they make great panini (see Apple Cheddar Panino, page 94). To create variety, try different toppings. My personal favorite is a pinch of sea salt, poppy seeds, and sesame seeds. Onion and garlic bits or dried garlic powder are also good options. Sprinkle on the topping once you've poured the rounds onto the cookie sheets, and then bake.

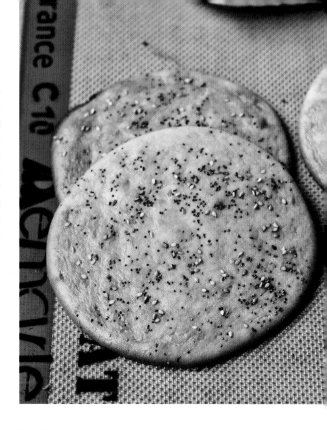

Makes 12 slices

  2½ cups blanched almond flour

  1 teaspoon baking soda

  1 cup SCD Yogurt (page 20)

  ¼ cup butter or ghee (page 23), melted

  3 large eggs

  2 tablespoons honey

  toppings, such as poppy seeds, sesame seeds, and coarse salt (optional)

1. Preheat your oven to 350°F/175°C. Line two or three (depending their size) baking sheets with nonstick baking mats, parchment paper, or other nonstick material.

2. Place all the ingredients except your toppings in a food processor; blend until creamy.

3. Pour 2-tablespoon batter circles onto the prepared baking sheets, leaving at least 2 inches between rounds. Use the back of a spoon to spread the batter out to the size you want, but don't make it too thin. If you want larger buns, use 3 or 4 tablespoons and don't spread them, because they'll spread sufficiently while baking.

4. Sprinkle with your chosen toppings and bake for 15 minutes, or until the rolls brown slightly on top. If you're making larger rolls, they'll take a few more minutes to brown and firm up sufficiently. Don't be afraid to go a little brown with these—that will make them firmer and add a tasty crunch at the edges.

5. Slide a knife or spatula under each roll and remove to a cooling rack. Let cool completely, seal, and store in the refrigerator for a week or so, or in the freezer for a few months.

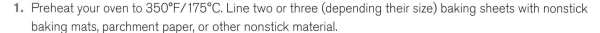

Nutrition per slice: *103 calories, 8 g fat, 6 g carbohydrate, 1 g fiber, 3 g protein*

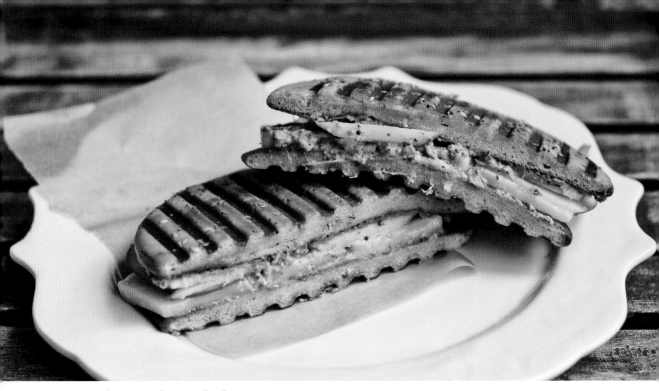

Apple Cheddar Panino

A panino is a pressed and toasted sandwich. Though it's often called a panini, with an "i" instead of an "o" at the end, that's actually the plural form of this popular sandwich. It's quite portable, which is one of the reasons I like it so much—toast, cool, and wrap, and you have a sandwich to go. The Sandwich Rounds on page 93 are excellent for panini, or you can use another bread recipe from this book.

This is one type of panino, but the possible combinations are endless. Put your favorite sandwich ingredients together, place the sandwich in the panini maker, and toast for a few minutes. It's that simple. You can make the sandwich either with a panini press, or with two frying pans. Just warm one pan over medium heat; butter the inside of that pan and the *bottom* of the second pan. Place the panino in the warm pan and press on it with the second pan for a few minutes. Once the first side is cooked, flip the panino and press again for a few minutes to cook the other side.

Makes 1 sandwich

2 Sandwich Rounds (page 93)

1 tablespoon stoneground mustard

½ cup shredded cheddar cheese (or a few thin slices)

½ apple, cored and thinly sliced (skin on or off)

1. Warm up your panini press.

2. Spread the mustard on the inside of each round, and then layer the cheese, apple, and prosciutto between the 2 sandwich rounds.

3. Place the sandwich in the panini press for about 3 minutes, or until the cheese begins to melt.

> **Nutrition per serving:** *510 calories, 24 g fat, 12 g carbohydrate, 3 g fiber, 16 g protein*

Blender Waffles

These are easy waffles—just place everything in a blender. Cashews lend a creamy flavor without the dairy, though you could substitute almonds, which have more fiber.

Makes 4 waffles

3 eggs

1 cup raw cashews or cashew pieces

⅓ cup dairy-free milk such as Almond Milk (page 13), Coconut Milk (page 15), or Cashew Milk (page 16)

3 tablespoons honey

3 tablespoons olive oil

3 tablespoons coconut flour

¼ teaspoon salt

¾ teaspoon baking soda

1. Preheat a waffle iron on a medium setting.

2. Add the eggs, cashews, milk, honey, and oil in a blender and blend until creamy and smooth.

3. Add the coconut flour, salt, and baking soda to the mixture and blend until smooth.

4. Pour about 2 tablespoons of batter into the waffle iron, or the amount your waffle iron calls for. You may have to experiment with the measurement the first few times to prevent the batter from overflowing.

5. Repeat with the remaining batter.

6. Serve warm. Store in the refrigerator for a week or so, or freeze for a few months.

Nutrition per waffle: *379 calories, 27 g fat, 25 g carbohydrate, 3 g fiber, 11 g protein*

Tips

◆ If you don't have dairy-free milk, use dairy-free yogurt or cashew cream.

◆ To make the waffles fluffier, add 1 teaspoon lemon juice to the milk or substitute the milk with yogurt.

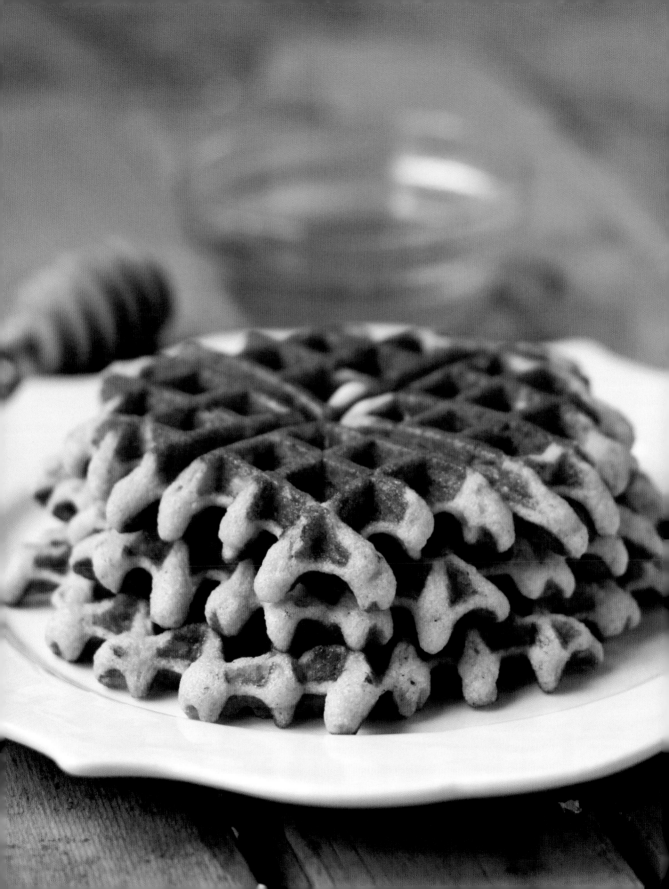

Almond Flour Waffles

I have fond memories of meeting my grandmother on Manhattan's Upper East Side for the best Belgian waffles in town. The narrow, hole-in-the-wall diner had the most enormous waffle makers I had ever seen.

The size of your waffles will depend on your waffle iron, too, and there are many to choose from. My latest model has a nonstick surface, but if you're not into that, there are waffle makers that have cast-iron surfaces. While I don't need to grease mine, I usually give it a quick rub of butter or oil before I begin. It's also a good idea to fully warm up the iron to ensure that the first waffle is just as good as the next. To crisp your cooked waffles, place them in a dehydrator or oven at 150°F/65°C for up to 30 minutes.

Makes 6 waffles

1 cup blanched almond flour (or other nut flour)

¼ teaspoon salt

¼ teaspoon baking soda

¼ teaspoon ground cinnamon (optional)

4 eggs

1 teaspoon vanilla extract

2 tablespoons honey

1. Preheat your waffle iron on a medium setting. Grease as needed, or according to the manufacturer's directions.

2. Place the almond flour, salt, baking soda, and cinnamon (if using) in a mixing bowl. Blend together using a whisk.

3. Add the eggs, vanilla, and honey and whisk until well blended.

4. Pour about ¼ cup batter into the heated waffle maker (more or less, depending on your waffle iron) and close the lid.

5. When the waffle is ready, transfer it to a plate and add your favorite topping. Seal and store any extra waffles in the refrigerator for a few days, or freeze them for up to a month or so.

> **Nutrition per waffle:** *98 calories, 6 g fat, 7 g carbohydrate, 1 g fiber, 5 g protein*

Almond and Coconut Flour Pancakes

Way back when I first whipped up a batch of pancakes, I was pretty satisfied and thought they had great texture and fluff. Fast forward to this recipe, where I've added an acidic ingredient to react with the baking soda to help the pancakes rise even more, giving you truly fluffy pancakes.

Makes 12 small pancakes

¼ cup coconut flour

1 cup almond flour

½ teaspoon baking soda

3 eggs

¼ cup yogurt

½ cup water

2 tablespoons honey

½ teaspoon vanilla extract

1 tablespoon sunflower oil or other mild-tasting oil, plus more for the skillet

pinch of salt (about ⅛ teaspoon)

1. Preheat a large skillet on medium-low heat.

2. Add all the ingredients in a food processor or blender and pulse for 10 seconds or so to combine.

3. Let the mixture sit for about a minute to let the coconut flour absorb the liquid.

4. Add 1 to 2 tablespoons of cooking oil to the hot skillet.

5. Spoon 1 to 2 tablespoons of batter per pancake into the skillet.

6. Cook the pancakes slowly on the first side, about 2 to 3 minutes or until bubbles start to appear on the top.

7. Once a pancake is starting to brown around the edges and the bottom, and can be flipped without the batter running, flip it to the other side to brown it for just another minute.

8. Repeat for the rest of the batter.

9. Store in the refrigerator for a week or so, or freeze for a few months.

> **Nutrition per pancake:** *65 calories, 4 g fat, 5 g carbohydrate, 1 g fiber, 3 g protein*

Tips

- To make these without yogurt and dairy-free, substitute the yogurt with ¼ cup coconut milk or other dairy-free milk with 1 teaspoon lemon juice.

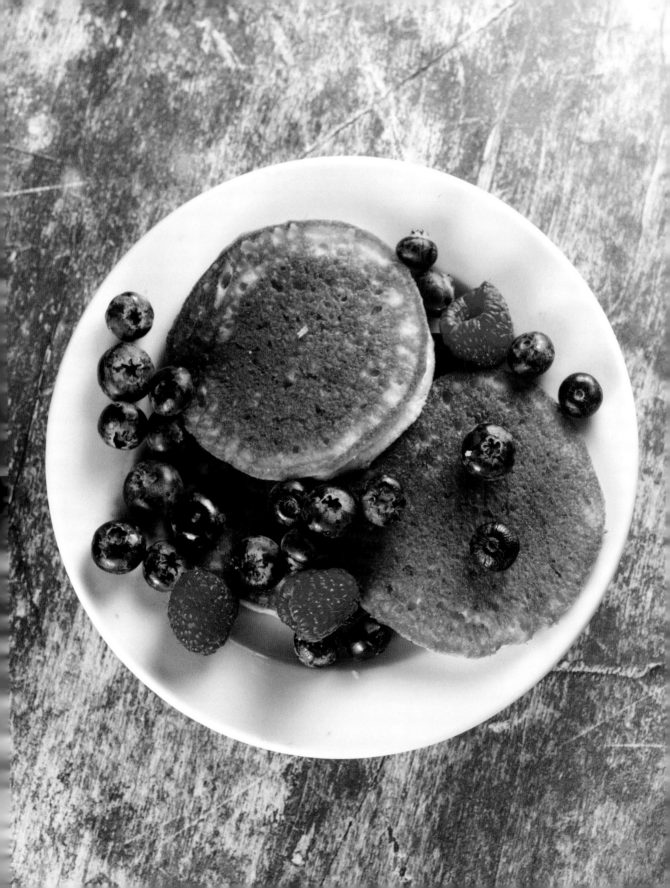

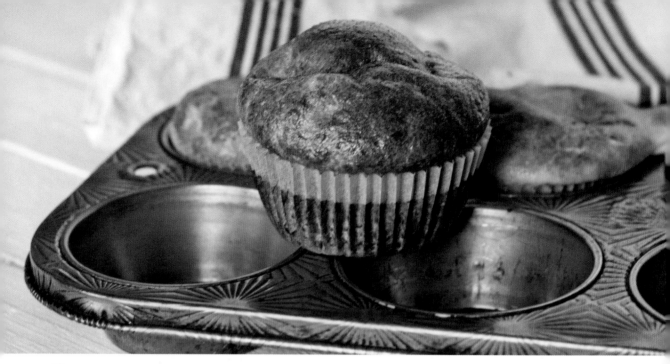

Popovers

These popovers, made with coconut flour and dairy-free milk, are delightfully light on their own. You can add herbs and spices to give these an added flavor, and top the popovers with grated Parmesan cheese, garlic powder, Parsley and Spinach Pesto (page 81), or minced fresh parsley. My personal favorite, though, is eating them plain, hot out of the oven, with a bit of butter and jam.

These are best eaten fresh from the oven, but you can store them at room temperature for a few hours if necessary. They'll deflate after several minutes, but they'll still look and taste marvelous. If you add about a tablespoon of Crème Fraîche (page 24) or grated cheese to the batter, the popovers will become denser and tend to hold their structure better after cooling. To bake these, use a muffin tin with nonstick muffin liners (see Product Sources, page 214), silicone baking cups, or a nonstick brioche or popover pan.

Makes 6 popovers

4 eggs	¼ teaspoon salt
½ cup coconut milk or other non-dairy milk	2 tablespoons coconut flour

1. Preheat your oven to 425°F/220°C. Prepare a muffin tin with nonstick liners or silicone cups or grease a brioche or popover pan, as needed.

2. In a bowl, whisk together all the ingredients until fully blended and a bit bubbly.

3. Fill the muffin or popover wells about ⅔ full with batter.

4. Bake for about 20 minutes, or until the popovers are brown on top. Let cool for a moment and then devour.

Nutrition per popover: *61 calories, 4 g fat, 2 g carbohydrate, 1 g fiber, 5 g protein*

Butter Biscuits

This is a very simple recipe that can easily be dressed up with seasonings or small chopped additions such as bacon bits, cheddar cheese, chives, and more. These are good as breakfast biscuits with scrambled eggs. I also use this recipe as a crust for Chicken Pot Pie (page 152).

Makes 6 biscuits

2½ cups blanched almond flour

½ teaspoon salt

½ teaspoon baking soda

2 eggs

¼ cup ghee (page 23) or unsalted butter, softened

1 tablespoon honey

1. In a bowl, combine the almond flour, salt, and baking soda; blend well using a fork.

2. In a separate bowl, whisk together the eggs, ghee or butter, and honey. Add to the dry ingredients and stir with a fork to blend thoroughly.

3. Roll the dough into a ball, wrap in waxed paper, and place in the freezer for about 10 minutes.

4. Preheat your oven to 350°F/175°C. Line a baking sheet with parchment paper or a nonstick baking mat.

5. Place the chilled dough between two pieces of parchment paper or other nonstick material and roll to a thickness of about 1 inch. Cut out biscuits using a cookie cutter. (Alternatively, you can roll small balls of dough in your hands, flatten them to about 1 inch thick, and shape into biscuits by hand.)

6. Place the biscuits on the prepared baking sheet and bake for about 12 minutes, or until they're browned on the outside and a toothpick inserted in the center comes out clean.

Nutrition per biscuit: *169 calories, 15 g fat, 6 g carbohydrate, 1 g fiber, 5 g protein.*

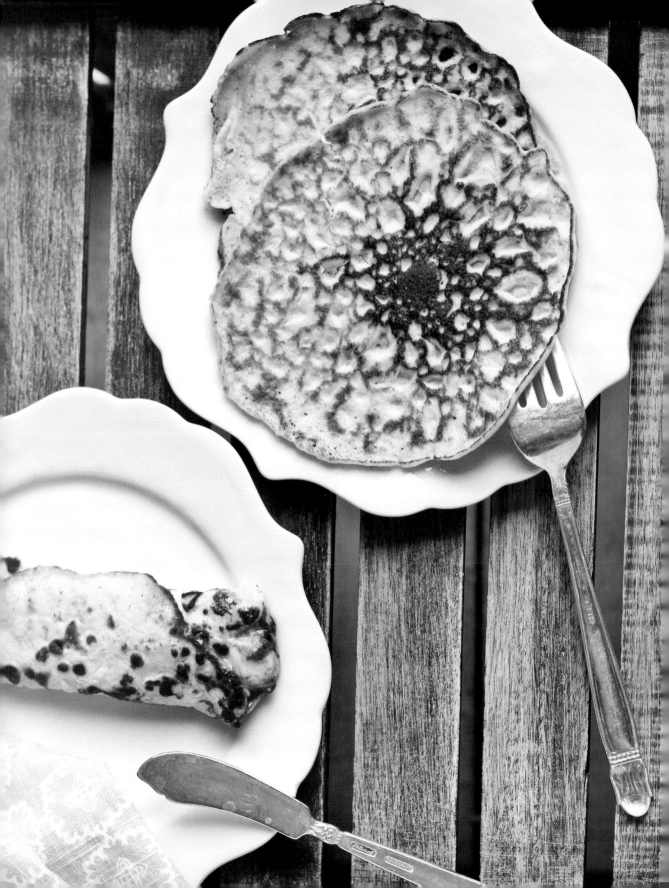

Crêpes

A crêpe is a very thin pancake that can be filled with just about anything sweet or savory. This recipe is simple in nature and easy to prepare. Just whisk together the ingredients and prepare a hot skillet.

Filling ideas for your crêpes include yogurt and fruit, Roasted Ratatouille (page 133), jam and cheese, and ham and egg scramble.

Makes 6 crêpes

2 eggs

2 tablespoons butter, ghee (page 23), or coconut oil, melted, plus more for the skillet

1 teaspoon honey

⅓ cup dairy-free milk (almond or other)

2 tablespoons coconut flour

⅛ teaspoon salt

1. In a bowl, whisk together the eggs, 2 tablespoons butter, ghee, or oil, honey, and milk.

2. Add the coconut flour and salt and whisk until well blended. Let the batter sit for a few minutes so the coconut flour can absorb the moisture.

3. Heat a skillet over medium heat and add about 1 tablespoon butter or oil.

4. Once the skillet is warm, pour in about 2 tablespoons batter to make a 4 to 5-inch crêpe and tilt the pan to allow the batter to spread across skillet in the shape of a circle.

5. After a few minutes, when the edges and bottom are starting to brown and you can easily slip a spatula underneath, flip the crêpe to the other side. Cook another minute or so on the other side, or until it is slightly browned.

6. Transfer the cooked crêpe onto a plate and repeat with the rest of the batter. Place waxed paper or paper towels between the crêpes on the plate to keep them from sticking.

7. To serve, fold or roll the crêpes around your chosen filling. Or, cover the unfilled crêpes and store in the refrigerator for up to a week or so.

> **Nutrition per crêpe:** *101 calories, 7 g fat, 6 g carbohydrate, 1 g fiber, 3 g protein*

Almond Brioche

This moist, brioche-style bread can be baked either as a loaf or as rolls. The rolls will bake much faster than the bread, so keep that in mind.

Makes 10 servings

2½ cups blanched almond flour

1 teaspoon baking soda

1 cup SCD Yogurt (page 20)

¼ cup butter or ghee (page 23), melted

3 large eggs

2 tablespoons honey

1. Preheat your oven to 350°F/175°C. Line a loaf pan with parchment paper if you're making bread, or insert nonstick liners in the wells of a standard-size muffin tin (or use silicone muffin cups). For the loaf pan, you can line the bottom of the pan and grease the sides, or insert the parchment paper to completely cover the inside.

2. Place all the ingredients in the bowl of a food processor. Blend until the mixture is creamy.

3. Pour the batter into the prepared loaf pan, or fill the muffin cups about ⅔ full.

4. Bake the bread for 50 minutes, or until a long toothpick or wooden skewer comes out clean; the top will be brown and have a hard crust. Bake the rolls for 12 minutes, or until they've browned slightly on top.

5. Let cool for a few minutes. Serve, or seal and store at room temperature for a few days, in the refrigerator for a week or so, or in the freezer for a few months.

> **Nutrition per serving:** *124 calories, 10 g fat, 7 g carbohydrate, 1 g fiber, 4 g protein*

Pumpkin Bread

After many requests, I started experimenting with pumpkin bread recipes. As a result, there are at least three baked pumpkin goodies on my website. But this one remains one of my favorites because of its flavor and moistness. It's almost a cake.

I usually use homemade squash puree in this recipe, but you can used canned as well. To make your own roasted pumpkin or squash puree, see page 130.

Makes 10 servings

¾ teaspoon baking soda

½ teaspoon salt

½ teaspoon ground nutmeg

½ teaspoon ground cinnamon

½ teaspoon ground cloves

½ teaspoon ground ginger

2 cups blanched almond flour

1 cup squash or pumpkin puree (homemade or canned)

1 cup honey

2 eggs

1. Preheat your oven to 350°F/175°C. Grease a loaf pan, about 8 x 5 inches.

2. In a bowl, combine all the dry ingredients in the order listed (baking soda through almond flour); blend well.

3. In a separate bowl, combine the squash puree, honey, and eggs, blending thoroughly.

4. Combine the wet and dry ingredients and blend well.

5. Scoop the batter into the prepared pan and bake for 60 minutes, or until the outside is brown and a toothpick inserted in the center comes out clean. The darker you go, the better it tastes, in my opinion. It might take more or less time, depending on how moist your puree is.

6. Cover and store at room temperature for a few days, in the refrigerator for a few weeks, or in the freezer for a few months.

Nutrition per serving: *161 calories, 4 g fat, 32 g carbohydrate, 1 g fiber, 3 g protein*

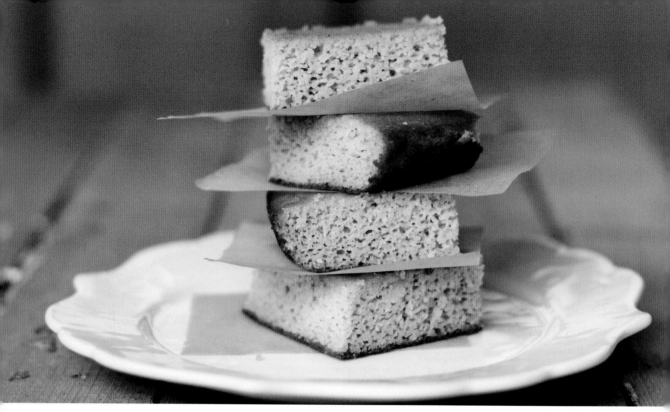

No-Corn Cornbread

Almond flour happens to make a fine base for "cornbread," even though it doesn't contain a single grain of cornmeal. Coconut flour lightens the texture, reduces the amount of nut flour needed, and adds a boost of good fiber.

This is a slightly sweet, slightly salty, slightly buttery version of cornbread—the basic kind. It's the softer, cakelike kind, not grainy, unless you use a grainier grind of almond or coconut flour. Feel free to add minced jalapeno, chili powder, chives, or grated Cheddar to make the bread savory. Or if you like it sweeter, add 1 tablespoon more honey. Or just bake the basic cornbread, let it cool for a minute, slice it into squares, and serve it with a hot bowl of your favorite chili or soup.

Baked in an 8 x 8-inch baking pan, this bread gets about 1 inch thick. For thicker bread, use a smaller pan or double the recipe and use a larger pan (about 9 x 12-inch size).

Makes 12 squares

½ cup blanched almond flour

¼ cup coconut flour

¼ teaspoon salt

¼ teaspoon baking soda

3 eggs

¼ cup unsalted butter, melted

2 tablespoons honey

½ cup almond milk (or other dairy-free milk or SCD Yogurt, page 20)

1. Preheat your oven to 325°F/165°C. Line the bottom of a baking pan (8 x 8-inch size or smaller) with parchment paper or other nonstick material, or grease well.

2. Blend the almond and coconut flours, salt, and baking soda in a bowl. (I use a stand mixer and mixing bowl.)

3. Add the eggs, butter, honey, and almond milk. Blend well.

4. Pour the batter into the prepared pan and bake for 20 minutes, or until a toothpick inserted in the center comes out clean.

5. Let cool briefly on a wire rack and then cut into squares. The bread can be sealed and stored in the refrigerator for a week or so, or frozen for a few months.

Nutrition per square: *82 calories, 6 g fat, 5 g carbohydrate, 1 g fiber, 2 g protein*

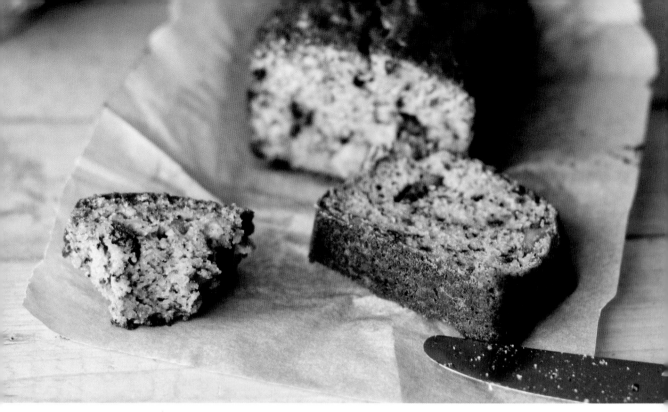

Banana Bread

This is one of those recipes that grew out of a few other recipes and became one of the most reliable staples for my family, for friends, for my website readers—and for good reason. It's unbreakable, and it tastes great. This recipe is easy to multiply. I always double it, and I triple it if I'm planning to give a loaf away.

You can use a 5 x 8-inch pan for this, but I usually use a smaller 3½ x 7½-inch loaf pan for this bread. The loaf will have a flat top in the larger pan, and it will be taller in a smaller loaf pan. If you want the loaf to lift out of the pan easily, line the inside with parchment paper. Otherwise just oil or butter it.

Makes 10 servings

¾ teaspoon baking soda

½ teaspoon sea salt

¾ cup almond flour

¼ cup coconut flour

2 tablespoons olive oil (or other cooking oil)

3 eggs

2 very ripe bananas, mashed (about 1 cup)

¼ cup honey

½ cup chopped walnuts (optional)

1. Preheat your oven to 350°F/175°C. Oil or butter a 5 x 8-inch or smaller loaf pan, or cover the bottom of sides of the pan with parchment paper if you want to be able to lift the loaf out of the pan.

2. Using a whisk or fork, blend the baking soda, salt, and flours in a bowl.

3. In a separate bowl, mix together the oil, eggs, mashed bananas, and honey. Combine the blended wet ingredients with the dry ingredients. I use an electric mixer to ensure that the batter is well blended.

4. Pour the batter into the prepared pan. Bake for 40 minutes, or until the sides and top are browned and a toothpick inserted in the middle comes out clean.

5. Let cool in the pan or on a cooling rack, and slice. To store, cover and refrigerate for up to a few weeks, or freeze for a month or so.

Nutrition per serving: *119 calories, 6 g fat, 13 g carbohydrate, 1 g fiber, 3 g protein*

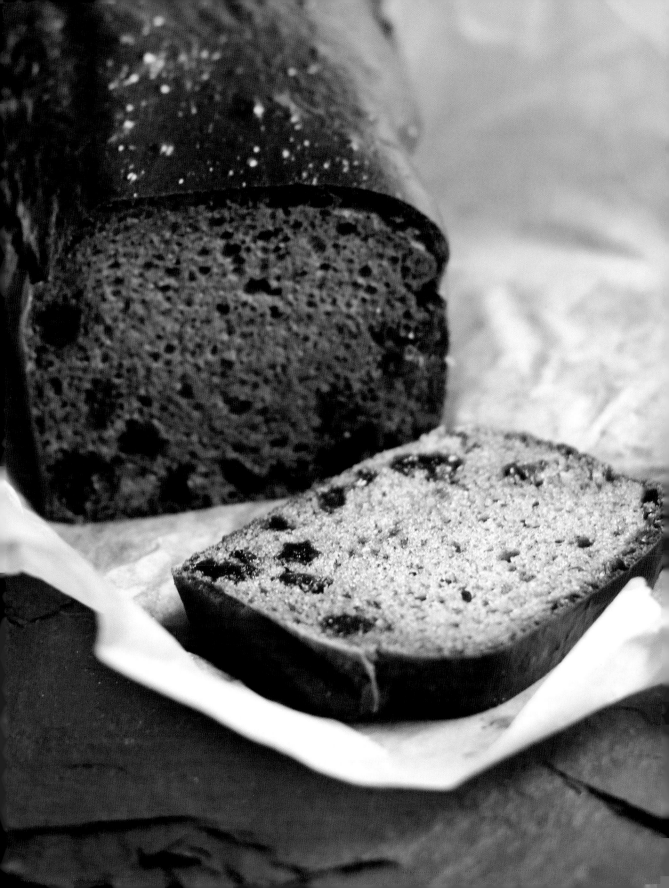

Cinnamon Raisin Bread

This bread recipe uses both almond butter and almond flour. The creamy butter makes it soft, and honey makes it slightly sweet. You can use either raw or roasted almond butter with this recipe.

I use a good amount of raisins because I love them, but you could easily reduce the amount to ½ cup if you prefer just a few raisins in each slice. The raisins tend to be a bit heavier than the batter and will gravitate toward the bottom of the bread. To counteract this, I add half the raisins to the batter, then sprinkle the rest over the batter once it's poured into the baking pan.

Makes 10 servings

¾ cup smooth almond butter

4 eggs

2 tablespoons honey

¼ cup blanched almond flour

½ teaspoon salt

½ teaspoon baking soda

1 teaspoon ground cinnamon

1 cup raisins

1. Preheat your oven to 350°F/175°C. Line a loaf pan with parchment paper. I either line the entire pan, or at least the bottom and then grease the sides. I use a smaller pan, about 4 x 7 inches, but any pan around this size will work, since the loaf does rise.

2. Using either a spatula or mixer, blend the almond butter, eggs, and honey in a large bowl until creamy.

3. In a separate bowl, blend the almond flour, salt, baking soda, and cinnamon together. Add the dry mix to the almond butter batter and blend well.

4. Stir half of the raisins into the batter, blending well.

5. Pour the batter into the prepared baking pan and then sprinkle the rest of the raisins over the top. Use a spoon or spatula to press them into the batter.

6. Bake for 45 minutes, or until a long toothpick or wooden skewer inserted all the way into the center comes out clean. Make sure the very bottom of the loaf is baked.

7. Let cool and slice. Seal and store in the refrigerator for a week or so, or freeze for up to a few months.

Nutrition per serving: *161 calories, 13 g fat, 39 g carbohydrate, 4 g fiber, 8 g protein*

English Muffin

When you're craving bread, use this quick and easy recipe to whip up an English muffin in a microwave. It's not identical to one made with all-purpose flour, but it's pretty darn close. While the muffin is pretty basic, it becomes a meal when toasted, buttered, and piled with eggs, spinach, and other great toppings.

Makes 3 servings

¼ cup blanched almond flour

1 tablespoon coconut flour

⅛ teaspoon baking soda

⅛ teaspoon salt

1 large egg white

½ teaspoon oil

1 tablespoon warm water

1. Add the flours, baking soda, and salt to a 3½-inch ramekin or small microwave-safe bowl. Mix well with a fork.

2. Add the egg white, oil, and water, and mix well.

3. Even out the batter on the top with a fork, spoon, or your fingers.

4. Microwave on high for 2 minutes.

5. Cool for a moment, and then turn the ramekin upside down to remove the muffin.

6. Cut the muffin into 3 slices and toast.

7. Add butter, jam, or other toppings.

Nutrition per serving: *82 calories, 7 g fat, 3 g carbohydrate, 2 g fiber, 4 g protein*

Tips

◆ I use a 3½-inch ramekin, which holds about 4 ounces of liquid and yields 3 slices. Depending on the diameter of your baking dish, you may get just 2 slices.

◆ To produce a more crumbly texture, you can bake the muffin in a conventional oven. Generously oil the inside of a 3½-inch ramekin and bake in a preheated oven at 400°F/200°C for 15 minutes. You may need to slide a knife along the sides to wiggle the muffin out.

◆ If you want to purchase a container of egg whites instead of using a whole egg and having a leftover yolk, 1 large egg white is equal to 2 tablespoons of egg white.

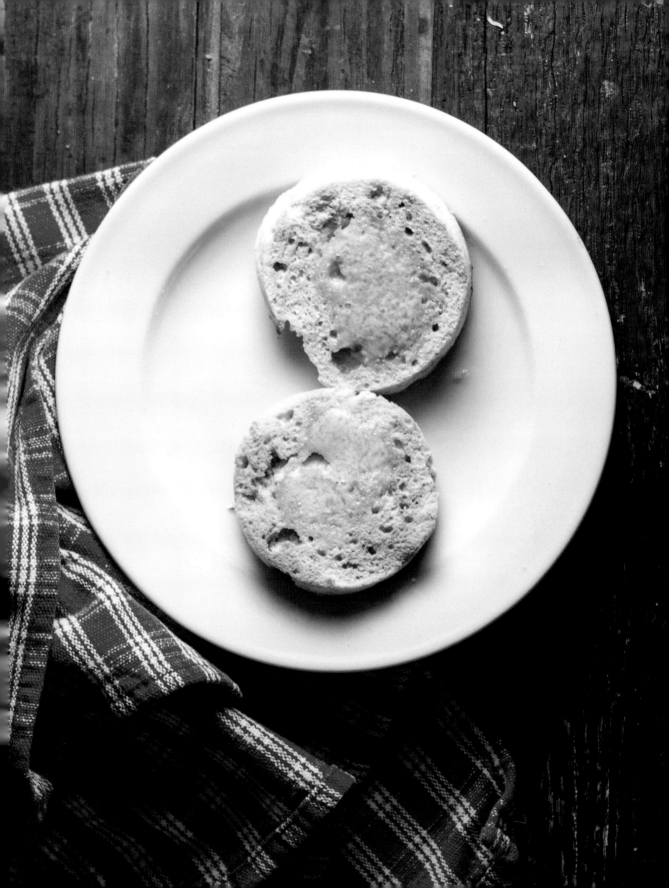

Cinnamon Raisin English Muffin

Add cinnamon, honey, and raisins to the English Muffin recipe on page 112 for a slightly sweeter version that's a bit moister in texture.

Makes 3 servings

¼ cup blanched almond flour

1 tablespoon coconut flour

⅛ teaspoon baking soda

⅛ teaspoon salt

¼ teaspoon ground cinnamon

1 large egg white

½ teaspoon oil

½ teaspoon honey

1 tablespoon warm water

1. Add the flours, baking soda, salt, and cinnamon to a 3½-inch ramekin or microwave-safe bowl. Mix well with a fork.

2. Add the egg white, oil, honey, and water, and mix well.

3. Even out the batter on the top with a fork, spoon, or your fingers.

4. Microwave on high for 2 minutes.

5. Cool for a moment, and then turn the ramekin upside down to slide the muffin out.

6. Slice the muffin into 3 slices and toast each slice.

7. Add butter, jam, or other toppings.

> **Nutrition per serving:** *91 calories, 7 g fat, 6 g carbohydrate, 2 g fiber, 4 g protein*

Tips

♦ I use a 3½-inch ramekin, which holds about 4 ounces of liquid and yields 3 slices. Depending on the diameter of your baking dish, you may get just 2 slices.

♦ To produce a more crumbly texture, you can bake the muffin in a conventional oven. Generously oil the inside of a 3½-inch ramekin or bowl and bake in a preheated oven at 400°F/200°C for 15 minutes. You may need to slide a knife along the sides to wiggle it out.

Cinnamon Bun Muffins

This is a well-loved recipe from my website, and I actually have two versions: this one using coconut flour and another using almond flour. Both are good, but the coconut flour recipe seems to be just a bit more popular. I couldn't imagine not including it in this book.

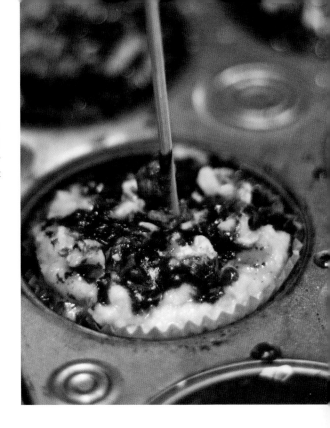

Makes 8 muffins

MUFFINS

½ cup coconut flour

¼ teaspoon baking soda

¼ teaspoon sea salt

4 eggs

⅓ cup SCD Yogurt (page 20) or dairy-free milk

½ cup honey

CINNAMON TOPPING

2 tablespoons ground cinnamon

¼ cup honey

2 tablespoons unsalted butter, ghee (page 23), or coconut oil, melted

1. Preheat your oven to 350°F/175°C. Insert nonstick muffin liners into the wells of a muffin tin.

2. For the muffins, combine the coconut flour, baking soda, and salt in a bowl and blend well.

3. Add the eggs, yogurt, and honey, using an electric mixer or blending well with a whisk. Make sure no clumps of flour remain.

4. Fill the muffin liners about ¾ full with batter.

5. In a small bowl, blend the topping ingredients together. Drip topping over each muffin. Some will sink into the batter, and you can use a toothpick to poke topping into the batter to spread it around.

6. Bake for about 20 minutes, or until a toothpick inserted in the center of a muffin comes out clean. Serve warm; or let cool, cover, and store for a few days at room temperature or for a week or so in the refrigerator.

Nutrition per muffin: *226 calories, 6 g fat, 38 g carbohydrate, 3 g fiber, 7 g protein*

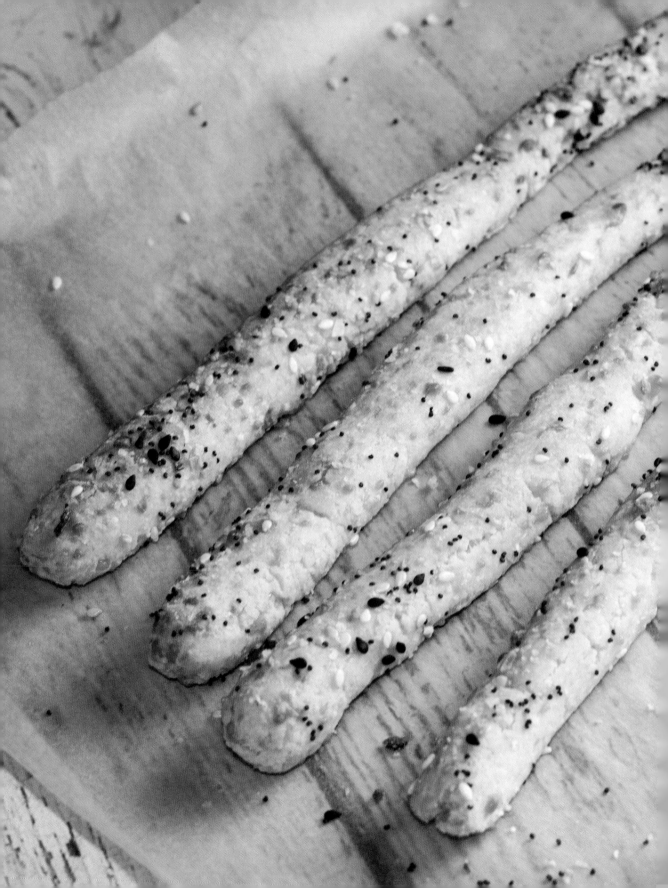

Breadsticks

Breadsticks are a fun addition to a salad or soup, or a satisfying snack with a side of Classic Marinara Sauce (page 78). You can double or even triple this recipe to feed a crowd, and it's likely you'll want more of these even without a crowd.

Makes 4 breadsticks

1 cup almond flour

1 cup grated Parmesan cheese (or any hard cheese)

1 egg

2 tablespoons toppings such as sesame seeds, poppy seeds, and salt (optional)

1. Preheat your oven to 350°F/190°C. Line a baking sheet with parchment paper or a nonstick baking mat.

2. Add the almond flour, cheese, and egg to a large bowl and blend until a soft dough forms.

3. Divide the dough into 4 balls. Use your hands to roll each ball into the shape of a breadstick then roll in the topping, if using. Place on the prepared baking sheet.

4. Bake the breadsticks for 15 minutes until lightly golden.

5. Cool for a few minutes. Store in the refrigerator for a few weeks or the freezer for a few months.

Nutrition per breadstick: *163 calories, 12 g fat, 5 g carbohydrate, 1 g fiber, 10 g protein*

Tortillas

These easy-to-make tortillas can be pulled out of the refrigerator at a moment's notice for a quick meal or snack. Make sure to place wax or parchment paper between the tortillas to make them easy to separate.

You can top these with just about anything, including marinated grilled veggies, fish, and chicken. You can also use them to make baked enchiladas and burritos. One of my favorite ways to use them is to create Fish Tacos (page 174). These modest-sized tacos are easier to fold (less fragile) than larger ones.

Makes 6 servings

⅔ cup egg whites (about 4 large egg whites)

2 tablespoons butter, ghee (page 23), or coconut oil, melted, plus more for the skillet

¼ cup dairy-free milk (almond or coconut works well)

1 tablespoon fresh lime juice

2 tablespoons coconut flour

¼ teaspoon ground cumin

¼ teaspoon salt

1. In a bowl, whisk together the egg whites, 2 tablespoons butter (or ghee or oil), milk, and lime juice.

2. Add the coconut flour, cumin, and salt; whisk until well blended. Let the batter sit for a few minutes so the coconut flour can absorb the moisture.

3. Heat a skillet over medium heat and add about 1 tablespoon butter or oil.

4. Once the skillet is warm, pour in about 2 tablespoons batter to make a 4 to 5-inch tortilla.

5. After a few minutes, when the edges and bottom are starting to brown and you can easily slip a spatula underneath, flip the tortilla to the other side.

6. Transfer the tortilla to a plate and repeat with the rest of the batter. Place waxed paper or parchment paper between the tortillas. Serve, or cover and store in the refrigerator for up to a week or so.

> **Nutrition per serving:** *80 calories, 4 g fat, 3 g carbohydrate, 1 g fiber, 3 g protein*

Quick Tips

- If you don't have enough egg whites, you can substitute 2 whole eggs for the whites.

- You can bake these tortillas, if you prefer. Preheat the oven to 400°F/200°C and line a baking sheet with parchment paper or a nonstick baking mat. Pour the batter in the shape of circles on the sheet and bake for 15 minutes. Use a spatula to flip them midway, at about 8 minutes.

Pizza Crust (Focaccia)

This recipe for a thick pizza crust has been on my website for quite a while and remains popular. It can be used with toppings or on its own as focaccia. You can easily substitute different types of nut flour and cheese.

The bottom of this cheesy crust gets nice and crunchy. You can serve this as either pizza or bread, with toppings or with flavored olive oils, and you can wrap it up and save it in the fridge or freezer, making it convenient for quick meals and snacks.

Makes 8 servings

2 cups blanched almond flour

¼ teaspoon each dried basil, dried oregano, and garlic powder (one or more are optional)

⅛ teaspoon sea salt

2 eggs

1 cup shredded cheese (cheddar, Parmesan, or a mix of soft and hard cheeses)

1 tablespoon olive oil

toppings, if desired

1. Preheat your oven to 350°F/175°C.

2. Blend the dry ingredients in a mixing bowl using a spatula or a mixer.

3. Add the eggs, cheese, and olive oil and blend well. Form into 2 or 4 dough balls, depending on how big you want your pizza pies.

4. On a nonstick baking mat or parchment paper, use your hands or a spatula to flatten 1 dough ball into a circular crust about ¼ inch thick, or thinner if you wish. I make individual pies, but a single big pie will work just as well. Lift the crusts and parchment paper or mat onto baking sheets.

5. Bake the crusts for about 15 minutes, or until they're as dark and firm as you want. The longer they stay in the oven, the crunchier the outer crust will be, top and bottom.

6. Add any toppings you like and bake for another 5 to 10 minutes, or remove from the oven and serve as flatbread slices or focaccia. To store, seal and refrigerate for a week or so, or freeze for about a month.

Nutrition per serving: *280 calories, 20 g fat, 3 g carbohydrate, 1 g fiber, 22 g protein*

Garlic Toasts

For this recipe, pick your favorite bread and combine it with your favorite olive oil, some garlic powder, and a dash of salt. For our family, this is a bit of heaven. Top these toasts with Tomato Bruschetta (page 43), or combine with a warm bowl of soup or Classic Marinara Sauce (page 78).

Makes 6 toasts

6 slices bread

2 tablespoons garlic powder

½ teaspoon salt

2 to 3 tablespoons olive oil

1. Preheat your oven to 350°F/175°C.

2. Place the bread slices on a baking sheet and sprinkle each slice with garlic powder and salt. Drizzle on some olive oil.

3. Toast the bread until it is brown around the edges.

4. Let cool and slice into triangles or rectangles. Store covered in the refrigerator for a week, or freeze for a few months.

> **Nutrition per toast:** *140 calories, 7 g fat, 17 g carbohydrate, 1 g fiber, 3 g protein*

Prescription Medication

It's okay to follow SCD while taking prescription drugs. Some people start out on medication and then follow SCD to slowly reduce their drug dependency, with the goal of transitioning to controlling their symptoms with just SCD. While you're probably hoping to avoid taking prescribed drugs, sometimes it may be necessary. Try not to feel defeated, but instead focus on eating well and learning to cook and prepare food that you like and need, and the rest will follow. It may be difficult to tell what's working and what's not, but you can figure that out as you go along, and as your body heals.

Vegetables and Mock Starches

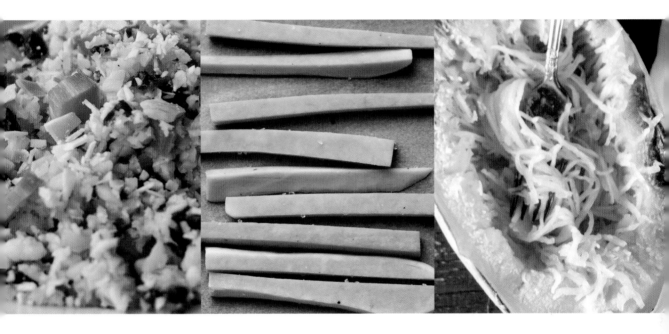

I'm a veggie lover, and I always have been. As a kid I loved all the green stuff—spinach, broccoli, Brussels sprouts, salads. I munched on whole sweet bell peppers as if I were grabbing an apple. I hope you'll find some green love, too, and incorporate vegetables into your daily meal planning. Some of the best sources of nutrients are green and bright-colored veggies, and the Roasted Ratatouille on page 133 fits that requirement easily. I keep a huge supply of it in my refrigerator so that I always have the makings of a quick bruschetta or sandwich.

Zucchini Noodles

Instantly turn a zucchini into a bed of noodles (also known as zoodles) resembling spaghetti. There are several ways to create the noodles: The easiest option is to use a spiralizer tool, but you can also use a mandolin or a julienne peeler. You can stir fry in a skillet, use in a spaghetti bake, toss with pesto and your choice of veggies, or simply eat raw. I've also heated them on high for 30 seconds in a microwave oven.

Makes 4 servings

4 medium zucchinis

Trim the stems off then spiralize each zucchini. I leave the green skin on, but feel free to remove it, if you prefer.

Nutrition per serving: 33 calories, 0 g fat, 6 g carbohydrate, 2 g fiber, 2 g protein

Simple Quiche

Here's a very easy recipe for a quiche that can be made with or without a crust. In fact, I kind of like it without a crust, because that frees me up to have just one step in the process. If you prefer a crust, use the Almond Tart Crust.

Feel free to adjust the ingredients—just keep the general ratio the same. It's really hard to mess this one up, so use whatever you have on hand. This is also convenient to have for ongoing leftovers as a snack, lunch, or breakfast. Reheat at 375°F/190°C for 5 minutes or so.

Makes 8 servings

8 eggs, lightly beaten

1 cup (about 4 ounces) shredded cheese (Cheddar or other aged cheese)

1 cup SCD Yogurt (page 20) or a soft cheese

1 cup chopped veggies or cured meat (greens, bell peppers, ham, raw bacon)

2 green onions, chopped

⅛ teaspoon salt

¼ cup chopped jalapeno chiles (optional; if you like heat, don't remove the seeds)

1 prepared Almond Tart Crust (page 123; optional)

1. Preheat your oven to 375°F/190°C.

2. Mix all the filling ingredients together in a big bowl.

3. Pour the mixture into an 8-inch baking pan or a prepared tart crust, if you're using one. Bake for about 25 minutes, or until the top begins to brown and the center is firm.

4. Cool for a few minutes, cut into 8 slices, and serve warm, or store in the refrigerator, covered, for up to a week.

Nutrition per serving: 196 calories, 16 g fat, 10 g carbohydrate, 3 g fiber, 15 g protein

Almond Tart Crust

This tart crust can be used for quiches and savory tarts, and the seasonings can be changed to suit your own preferences or what you have on hand. I sometimes add fresh chopped thyme or rosemary to the mix, or some dill and oregano when I'm including feta cheese in my tart filling.

Makes 8 servings

2 cups blanched almond flour or almond meal

½ teaspoon salt

¼ cup ghee (page 23), unsalted butter, or coconut oil, softened

1 tablespoon water

1 tablespoon chopped fresh herbs or 1 teaspoon dried herbs (optional)

1. Preheat your oven to 350°F/175°C.

2. Blend the almond flour or meal with the salt in a bowl.

3. Add the ghee, butter, or oil and the water, plus any herbs you're using. Blend until the dough is crumbly but sticks together when you press it with your fingers.

4. Press the dough into a tart pan or pie dish.

5. Bake for 10 minutes, or until the crust begins to brown slightly. Let cool for at least 10 minutes and then fill.

Nutrition per serving: *91 calories, 9 g fat, 2 g carbohydrate, 1 g fiber, 2 g protein*

Quick Tip

◆ This crust fills an 8-inch round tart pan or pie dish, or a 7 x 11-inch rectangular tart pan.

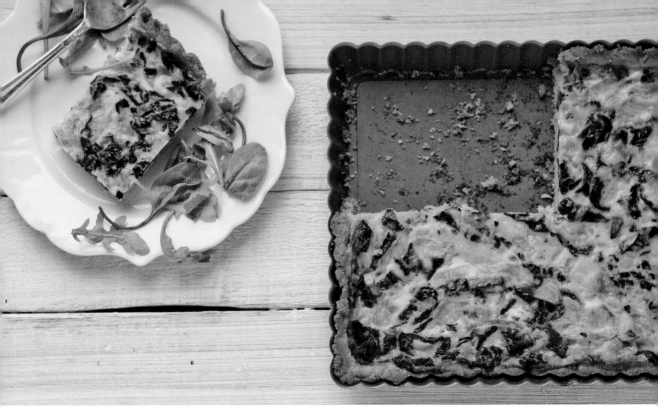

Kale Onion Tart

Caramelized onions lend wonderful flavor to any savory recipe, including vegetable tarts. You can take the time to fully caramelize the onions, or cut it short and only cook them for about 15 minutes. If you don't have kale, you can substitute other greens you may have on hand, such as spinach or chard. If you want more of a quiche from this recipe, just add a bit more salt and 2 more eggs. And if you want to leave out the cheese, you can substitute SCD Yogurt (page 20) or Crème Fraîche (page 24).

Makes 8 servings

2 tablespoons unsalted ghee (page 23) or other cooking oil (or a mix of both)

1 large onion (white or yellow), about 1 ½ cups finely diced

¼ teaspoon salt, divided

drizzle of honey (optional)

2 garlic cloves, peeled and minced

4 eggs, lightly beaten

3 cups torn kale, destemmed (from about 6 large leaves)

1 cup shredded Gruyère or other Swiss cheese (about 4 ounces)

1 prepared Almond Tart Crust (page 123), in a tart or pie pan

1. In a large skillet, heat the ghee or oil over medium heat.

2. Add the diced onions, sprinkle on ⅛ teaspoon salt, and cook for about 15 minutes, stirring occasionally, until the onions are translucent and beginning to brown. If you wish to fully caramelize the onions, cover the pan for the first 15 minutes, then uncover it, add a drizzle of honey, and cook for another 15 minutes, or until browned.

3. Add the garlic to the onion mixture and cook for a few more minutes.

4. Preheat your oven to 350°F/175°C.

5. Let the onion mixture cool in the skillet for a few minutes, then gently stir in the eggs, kale, shredded cheese, and ⅛ teaspoon salt.

6. Pour the filling into the prepared tart crust and bake for 20 minutes. Cool for a few minutes, cut into 8 pieces, and serve warm, or store in the refrigerator, covered, for up to a week.

Nutrition per serving: *290 calories, 19 g fat, 12 g carbohydrate, 5 g fiber, 14 g protein*

Squash Ribbon Noodles

These squash ribbons are a veggie replacement for regular noodles—not quite the same texture, but they go well with the right toppings. You can peel the squash into any width you prefer, but wide noodles are especially nice with heavier toppings such as tomato sauces, and in cheese-topped casseroles.

You'll want a vegetable peeler and skewers to create the squash ribbons. You can eat them raw or dry them out a bit as instructed below, using a dehydrator or your oven, and add a topping.

Makes 4 servings

4 medium zucchini or yellow squash (about 3 pounds)

about ½ tablespoon of olive oil, butter, or ghee (page 23; optional)

sea salt and pepper, to taste (optional)

1. Peel the skin off each zucchini (optional), keeping the stem top intact.

2. Place a skewer through the stem end to hold the zucchini in place while you use a vegetable peeler to cut wide ribbons of zucchini.

3. Place the zucchini ribbons on dehydrator sheets or a baking sheet lined with a nonstick baking mat (optional if you want to remove moisture from the noodles).

4. If you're using a dehydrator, set the temperature to about 120°F/50°C; dehydrate for about 5 minutes, or until the noodles have a texture you like and some of the moisture has been removed. If you're using an oven, set it as low as it will go and bake for about 5 minutes.

5. Place the squash noodles in a bowl and blend with a little olive oil (or butter or ghee), salt, and pepper to taste, if you wish. Alternatively, you might add Parsley and Spinach Pesto (page 81), grated Parmesan cheese, or Classic Marinara Sauce (page 78).

Nutrition per serving: *44 calories, 2 g fat, 6 g carbohydrate, 2 g fiber, 1 g protein*

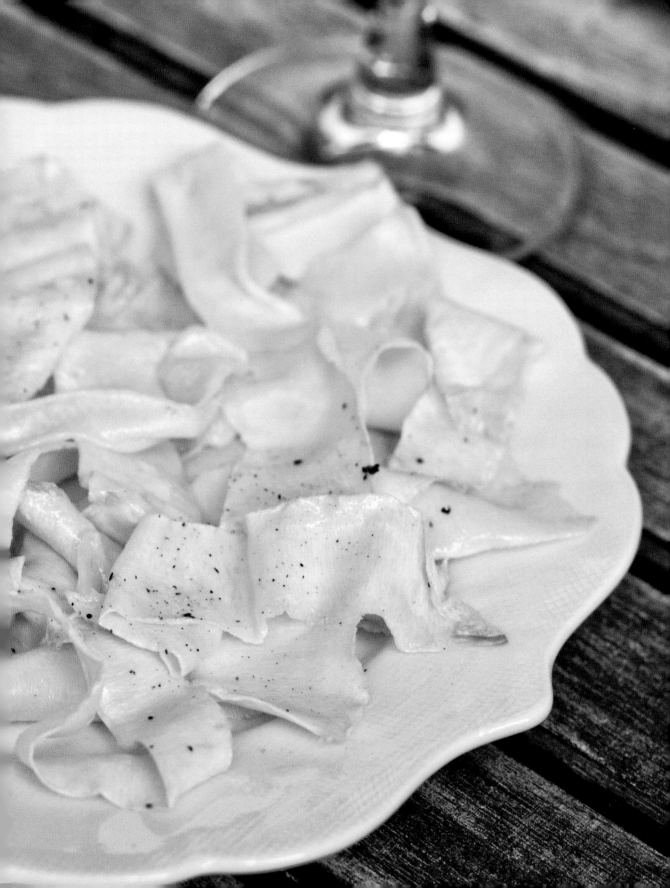

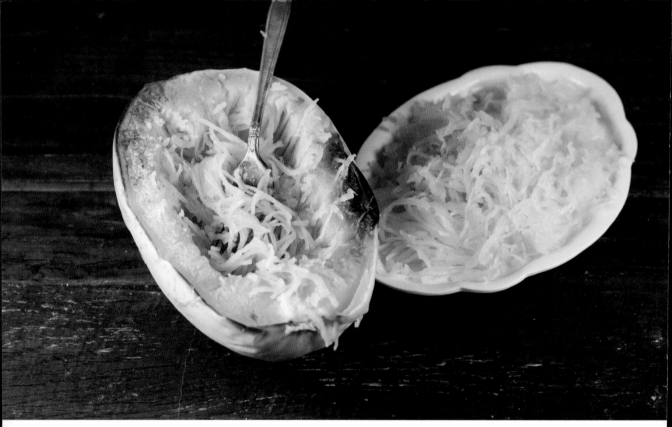

Spaghetti Squash

I love the simplicity of this squash. You're rewarded with a basic but versatile "spaghetti" without having to do any scraping, peeling, or other slicing tricks. Spaghetti squash does have a more neutral flavor than other squash varieties, which makes it perfect for dressing up with sauces, grated cheeses, flavored oils, and butters. Some of my favorite spaghetti squash toppings include meatballs and marinara sauce, Parmesan cheese and olive oil, pesto, or a pile of ratatouille with olive oil and grated Parmesan.

Like other winter squash, this one can be a bit challenging to cut open. If you find it difficult, try cracking the squash by making an indentation with a knife and then tapping the squash on a hard surface to crack it open. You may be tempted to cut your spaghetti squash lengthwise, which is fine, but the spaghetti strings actually run around the squash, not lengthwise. Cutting it into cross sections will give you longer spaghetti strings.

Makes 4 servings

    1 spaghetti squash (about 3 pounds)

    1 teaspoon ghee (page 23), coconut oil, or high-heat oil

1. Preheat your oven to 425°F/220°C.

2. Peel and cut the squash crosswise into 2 or 3 pieces. Scoop out the seeds, using a fork.

3. Lightly oil a baking sheet with the ghee or oil. Place the squash pieces, cut side down, on the baking sheet.

4. Bake for at least 30 minutes—or up to 40 minutes, depending on the size of your squash.

5. Let the squash cool for few minutes and then use a fork to scoop out the stringy pulp from the squash. Serve the "spaghetti" with your topping of choice.

Nutrition per serving: *62 calories, 0 g fat, 10 g carbohydrate, 2 g fiber, 1 g protein*

Roasted Butternut Squash (Pumpkin Puree)

Roasted squash puree is quite easy to make, though both canned and fresh work in my recipes. My preference is to use butternut squash, but pumpkin and other squash also work—they just aren't as sweet as butternut squash, generally.

The only disclaimer I would add is that fresh squash puree tends to be moister than the canned type, which can affect your recipe. (Bread made with fresh puree may be moister and take longer to bake.) I use a spoon to remove excess water when possible.

It can be quite treacherous cutting up some pumpkins and squash. If you can't cut without endangering a finger or other body part, try cracking your squash open by making a few strategic cuts around the outside and then prying it apart with your hands—or give it a gentle bounce on a hard surface.

Makes 4 (½-cup) servings

    1 butternut squash (about 2 pounds) or other winter squash

1. Preheat your oven to 350°F/175°C. Grease a rimmed baking sheet or pan.

2. Wash the squash and cut it in half (either lengthwise or crosswise works). Scoop out the seeds.

3. Place the halves cut side down on the prepared pan. Bake for 45 minutes, or until tender when pierced with a fork.

4. Let cool for several minutes and then scoop the flesh into the bowl of a food processor. Pulse until smooth.

5. Use a spoon to press out and remove excess water, and then your squash puree is ready to use. Or, you can seal and freeze it for up to a year.

Nutrition per serving: *102 calories, 0 g fat, 27 g carbohydrate, 5 g fiber, 2 g protein*

Garlic Mashed "Potatoes"

This is a classic recipe for mashed "potatoes"—also known as mashed roasted cauliflower. While you can find this recipe dressed up in various ways all over the Internet, I thought I'd also include it here, since it's such a fine side dish.

Makes 4 servings

1 large cauliflower head

1 garlic clove, minced

¼ teaspoon salt

2 tablespoons melted ghee (page 23) or other cooking oil

1 to 2 cups warm water or dairy-free milk

1. Preheat your oven to 400°F/200°C.

2. Cut the cauliflower into bite-size pieces and place them in a bowl. Add the garlic, salt, and ghee or oil and stir to fully coat the cauliflower.

3. Place the cauliflower on a baking sheet and bake for about 20 minutes, or until the cauliflower is browning around the edges.

4. Let the cauliflower cool for a few minutes and then transfer it to a blender or food processor. Slowly blend in water or milk until the mashed cauliflower mixture is the consistency you like.

Nutrition per serving: *109 calories, 8 g fat, 20 g carbohydrate, 7 g fiber, 6 g protein*

Soothing the Soul

Your mind plays an important role in your physical well-being. Here are a few ideas for soothing your soul: listen to music, go on a walk, take a nap, do some stretching or yoga, meditate, read a book, play a game, watch a movie, talk to a friend, laugh as much as possible. Eliminate or reduce things that bring stress to your life. Give yourself permission to lie low, listen to soothing music, meditate, and indulge in what makes you feel happy.

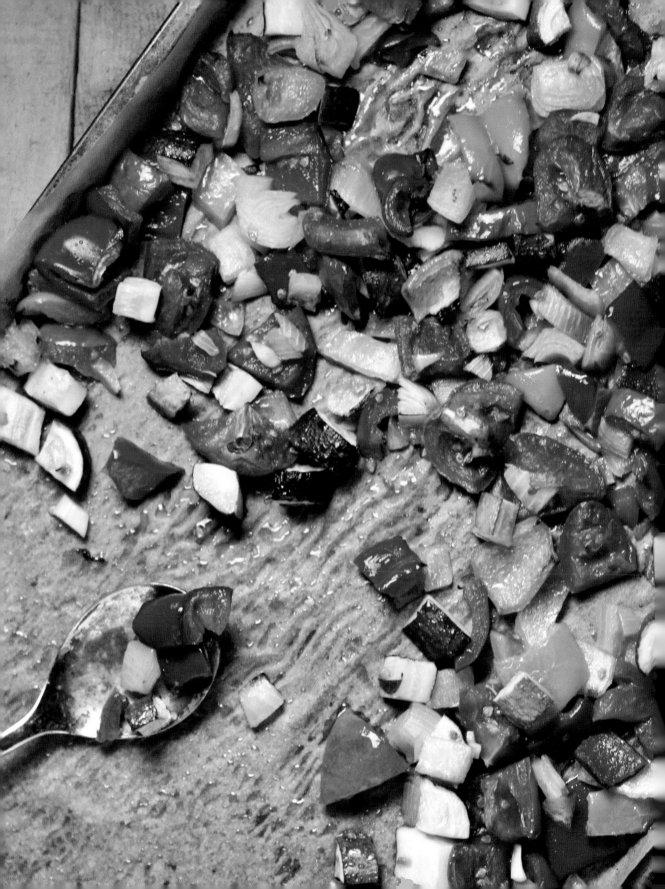

Roasted Ratatouille

This is my go-to veggie comfort dish, and I almost always have a container of it in the refrigerator, ready at a moment's notice. Just give me a big bowl of this ratatouille, sprinkled generously with Parmesan cheese, and I'm a happy camper. I make a large batch and eat it for days, adding it to quiches and eggs or spreading it on slices of toast to make bruschetta. Ratatouille is so open to change-ups, meaning you can add just about any vegetable, make substitutions, and season to your liking. It's kind of like regular roasted vegetables, except that you don't want to spread out the veggies on the baking sheets. Instead, you want them piled a bit on top of each other so they steam together a bit.

Traditional ratatouille includes eggplant and tomatoes, but if you are avoiding these you can substitute mushrooms and other seasonal veggies that will roast in about 40 minutes.

Makes 4 servings

2 large zucchini

1 medium eggplant, diced into bite-size pieces (optional)

4 large plum tomatoes (about 1 pound)

2 large bell peppers (red and orange are my favorites)

1 large red onion (or other type), peeled and diced

¼ teaspoon salt, or to taste

4 garlic cloves, minced

3 tablespoons high-heat oil (or a mix of olive oil and high-heat oil)

1. Preheat your oven to 375°F/190°C. Line one or two rimmed baking sheets with nonstick baking mats or parchment paper.

2. Chop the zucchini, eggplant (if using), tomatoes, and peppers into bite-size pieces.

3. Toss all the ingredients together in a large bowl until the veggies are well coated with the oil. Spread the mixture out on the prepared baking sheets, allowing the veggies to pile onto each other a bit.

4. Bake for 40 minutes, or until the onions and tomatoes are soft. Serve either warm or at room temperature. Store in a covered container in the refrigerator for up to about a week.

> **Nutrition per serving:** *214 calories, 11 g fat, 28 g carbohydrate, 10 g fiber, 5 g protein*

Fresh Air and Exercise

Get outside every day for fresh air and sunlight. One hour of exposure to sunlight each day is the best source of vitamin D. Open up the windows in your house, and bring herbs and plants inside to freshen the air. Clean out air filters in furnaces and vacuum cleaners. Even in the winter, I keep a few windows cracked for fresh airflow. Find a happy balance with exercise that keeps you in shape without depleting the energy reserves you need for healing. Walking, running, sweating, stretching,

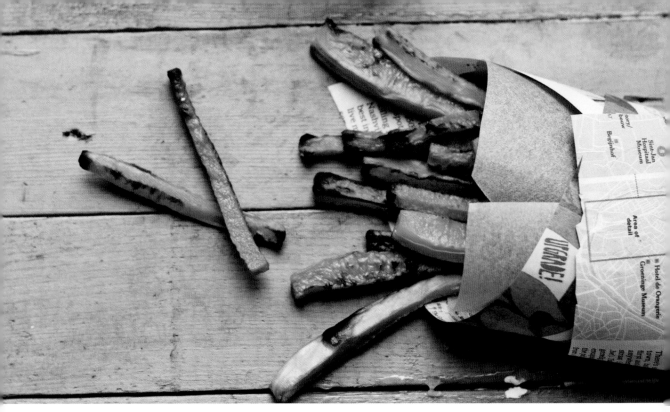

Sweet Fries

Here's a sweet fry that's full of vitamins A and C, with iron and calcium thrown in for good measure. I might even go so far as to say these can hold a candle to almost any fry. Well, I might be stretching it a bit here, but they are worth the effort and really tasty with homemade Simple Ketchup (page 80).

I suggest peeling the skin off before you cut the squash, because it's just easier. Then cut the squash either across the center or lengthwise, scoop out the seeds, and begin slicing for fries. Try to cut your fries all the same width and length, more or less, so they'll bake in about the same time.

Since the prep work takes a bit of time, you can peel and slice the squash ahead of time and store it in the refrigerator, or even freeze it. You can also dry the slices by leaving them out for a few hours before you plan to bake them. Frozen fries will take a bit longer to bake.

Makes 4 servings

1 butternut squash (about 3 pounds), peeled and sliced into fries (see note above)

½ teaspoon salt, plus more as needed

½ teaspoon high-heat oil (just enough to lightly coat each fry)

pepper, to taste

1. Place the cut fries in a bowl, sprinkle with the ½ teaspoon salt, and toss to coat.

2. Spread the fries out on a paper towel or kitchen cloth and let them sit for 30 minutes or so to sweat out moisture.

3. Preheat your oven to 425°F/220°C. Line a rimmed baking sheet with parchment paper.

4. Use a paper towel to wipe the moisture off the fries, then transfer them back to their bowl and blend with the oil.

5. Spread the fries out on the prepared baking sheet so they're not touching. Bake for 15 minutes on the first side, then flip them over and bake for another 7 minutes, or until crisped on the edges. If you want them crisped a bit more, turn off the oven and leave them in for about 5 more minutes.

6. Salt and pepper the fries to taste and serve hot. You can also reheat these for 5 minutes at 400°F/200°C.

Nutrition per serving: *21 calories, 1 g fat, 4 g carbohydrate, 1 g fiber, 0 g protein*

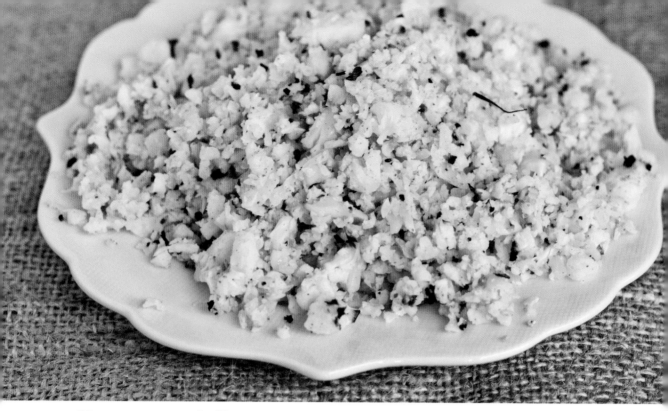

Yellow Cauliflower Rice

There's something about the appearance of yellow rice that almost allows me to taste all its flavors before it even reaches my mouth. It could be that yellow, buttery color that glows, thanks to the saffron and turmeric.

Saffron lends a unique flavor to the cauliflower in this recipe—but truth be told, when I don't have saffron the rice still tastes quite good. If you're not an onion fan, you can do without, but it does add an additional flavor dimension to this tasty rice.

Makes 4 servings

2 or 3 saffron threads

2 tablespoons cooking oil or ghee (page 23), divided

2 large cauliflower heads, cut into large pieces

¼ teaspoon ground turmeric

¼ teaspoon fine salt, plus more as needed

1 small white onion, finely diced

fish sauce (optional)

1. Preheat your oven to 400°F/200°C. Line a rimmed baking sheet with parchment paper or a nonstick baking mat.

2. Break the saffron threads into small pieces and place them in a large bowl. Add 1 tablespoon oil or ghee and set the bowl in a warm spot, such as next to a warm oven; leave for about 10 minutes.

3. Add the cauliflower, turmeric, and ¼ teaspoon salt to the saffron bowl and blend well to coat the cauliflower.

4. Spread the cauliflower onto the prepared baking sheet and bake for 15 minutes, or until the edges begin to brown and the cauliflower is tender when pierced with a fork.

5. Place the onions, fish sauce (optional), and remaining 1 tablespoon oil or ghee in a small skillet and cook over medium heat until the onions are translucent and starting to brown, about 8 minutes, stirring occasionally.

6. Let the cauliflower cool for a few minutes and then place it in a food processor to process into rice-size pieces, or chop finely by hand.

7. Combine the cauliflower rice with the onions and blend well. Add salt to taste.

Nutrition per serving: *156 calories, 7 g fat, 11 g carbohydrate, 3 g fiber, 3 g protein*

Orange Cauliflower Couscous

Here's a simple sweet "couscous" that pairs well with just about any grilled veggie or meat. I love it with fish that's also been flavored with citrus, such as the Citrus Tuna Kebabs (page 168). You could spice it up a bit by adding ginger and cinnamon, but I prefer this basic version most of the time. This dish also does well after being stored in the refrigerator for a few days, and brought to room temperature.

Makes 4 servings

¼ cup raisins or currants

1 large cauliflower head (or 2 small heads)

1 carrot, peeled

1 tablespoon melted ghee (page 23) or high-heat oil

⅜ teaspoon sea salt, divided, plus more as needed

2 tablespoons olive oil

1 tablespoon grated orange zest

4 tablespoons fresh orange juice

2 tablespoons crushed blanched almonds

orange slices, for garnish

1. Preheat your oven to 400°F/200°C.

2. Soak the raisins or currants in hot water (about the temperature of hot tap water) for about 5 minutes to soften them. Drain.

3. Chop up the cauliflower into small florets. Cut the carrot into a few long thin strips. In a bowl, mix the cauliflower and carrots with the 1 tablespoon melted ghee or oil and ¼ teaspoon sea salt.

4. Transfer the cauliflower and carrots to a rimmed baking sheet and roast for 15 minutes, or until they begin to brown at the edges. Let cool.

5. Separate the cooled carrots and cauliflower and place the cauliflower in the bowl of a food processor. Process until you have fine granules the size of couscous.

6. Chop the raisins and roasted carrots into fine pieces.

7. In a bowl, combine the cauliflower, 2 tablespoons olive oil, carrots, raisins, orange zest, orange juice, ⅛ teaspoon salt, and almonds. Add salt to taste.

8. Garnish with orange slices and serve warm or cold.

Nutrition per serving: *296 calories, 16 g fat, 37 g carbohydrate, 8 g fiber, 8 g protein*

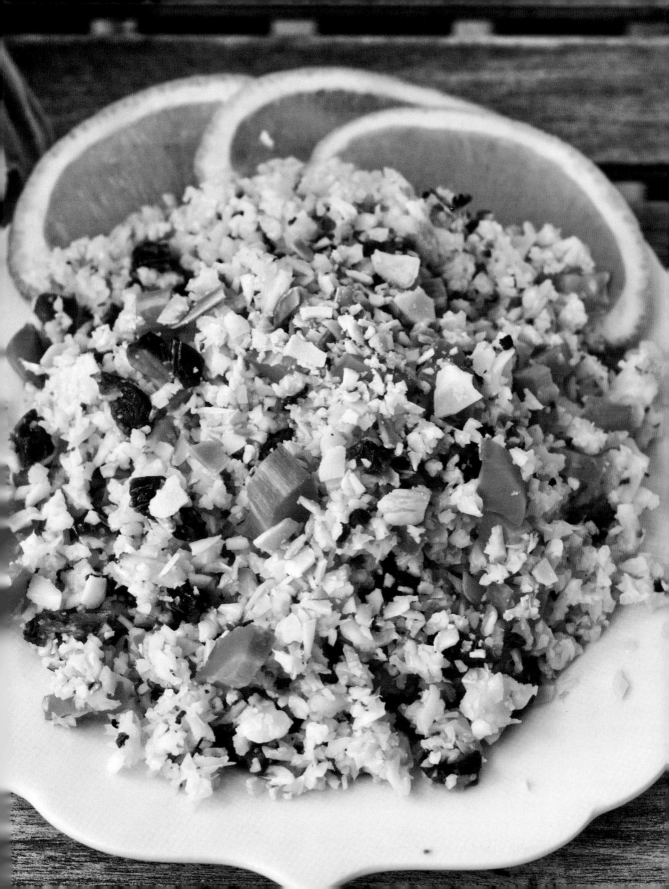

Roasted Cauliflower Rice

This is my favorite recipe for cauliflower rice, because the roasting locks in flavor and gives a texture that I find closest to actual rice. If you're sensitive to digesting roasted veggies, or to cauliflower itself, I'd recommend steaming your rice.

Makes 4 servings

2 large cauliflower heads, chopped into chunks

1 tablespoon cooking oil or ghee (page 23)

¼ teaspoon fine salt, plus more as needed

pepper, to taste

1. Preheat your oven to 400°F/200°C. Line a rimmed baking sheet with parchment paper or a nonstick baking mat.

2. Place the cauliflower, oil or ghee, and ¼ teaspoon salt in a bowl and mix well to coat the cauliflower.

3. Spread out the cauliflower on the prepared baking sheet and roast for 15 minutes, or until the edges begin to brown and the cauliflower is tender when pierced with a fork.

4. Let the cauliflower cool for a few minutes and then place it in the bowl of a food processor to process into rice-size pieces, or chop finely by hand.

Nutrition per serving: *135 calories, 4 g fat, 22 g carbohydrate, 11 g fiber, 8 g protein*

Emotional Support

Some who suffer from digestive conditions are lucky to have a support system built into their lives to help them get through the tough times. There are many sources for emotional support, but do seek out the help of friends, family, and others who can lend a hand. It might be a spouse, a friend, support groups, or just the unconditional love of a pet that helps you along. Don't discount this important part of healing.

Fried Cauliflower Rice

If you love Asian-style dishes that rely on soy sauce, I think you'll like this take on fried rice. Instead of soy sauce, I use Mock Soy Sauce—but don't sweat it if you don't have the sauce on hand. Several years ago, a friend who was born and raised in Japan brought me her version of fried rice, and it was delicious. I asked her what she seasoned it with and was surprised to hear she'd used only salt and pepper. Since then, I don't believe you have to have soy sauce for Asian foods to taste good. You just need to be a bit creative and take advantage of other seasonings available to you: ginger, salt, honey, vinegar, and—in this case—fish sauce.

Makes 4 servings

recipe for Roasted Cauliflower Rice (page 140)

2 tablespoons ghee (page 23) or cooking oil, divided

2 eggs, scrambled

1 cup finely diced peeled carrots (about 2 carrots)

1 cup finely diced celery

1 cup finely diced green onions

2 large garlic cloves, minced

Mock Soy Sauce (page 89), to taste

salt, to taste

1. Preheat your oven to 400°F/200°C and prepare the Roasted Cauliflower Rice according to the recipe instructions.

2. While the cauliflower is roasting, heat half of the ghee or oil in a wok or skillet over medium heat.

3. Add the eggs to the hot pan and either scramble them or cook them as a flat omelet and chop up at the end of cooking. Remove the eggs from the pan and set aside.

4. Add the rest of the ghee to the pan along with the carrots and celery. Cook for about 7 minutes, or until the vegetables begin to soften.

5. Add the garlic and onions to the pan and continue cooking for another 5 minutes. Add the roasted cauliflower and stir to blend well.

6. Add Mock Soy Sauce and salt to taste. Blend in the eggs and remove from the heat. Serve immediately, or cover and store in the refrigerator for up to a few days.

> **Nutrition per serving:** *187 calories, 9 g fat, 21 g carbohydrate, 8 g fiber, 10 g protein*

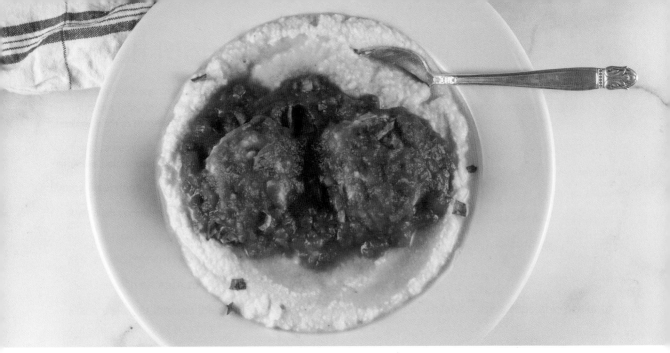

Cauliflower Polenta

Here's a corn-free take on polenta using the very versatile cauliflower. The vanilla of vegetables, cauliflower can take on many textures and flavors. Serve with meatballs, sautéed mushrooms, roasted vegetables, or dairy-free Creamed Spinach (page 144).

Makes 4 servings

1 large cauliflower head

4 tablespoons butter or ghee (page 23)

3 cups water

¼ teaspoon salt, plus more to taste

½ teaspoon ground turmeric

1 to 2 tablespoons grated Parmesan cheese (optional)

1. Chop the cauliflower into chunks and discard the leaves and stem bottom.

2. Pulse the cauliflower into small grain-like pieces—it should be more granular than riced cauliflower.

3. Preheat a frying pan over medium heat.

4. Add the cauliflower, butter or ghee, half the water, and salt, and stir until butter melts. Add the remaining 1½ cups water and simmer with a steady bubble for about 15 minutes or until the cauliflower is soft but not mushy. Add more water if you like a thinner consistency.

5. Turn off the heat and add the turmeric and more salt to taste or, if you prefer, 1 or 2 tablespoons grated Parmesan cheese.

6. Serve warm with your favorite toppings.

Nutrition per serving: *140 calories, 12 g fat, 8 g carbohydrate, 3 g fiber, 3 g protein*

Jeweled Cauliflower Rice

This mock rice dish is more than just another riced cauliflower recipe. It goes well with any savory protein, including Peri Peri Chicken (page 154) and Chicken Shawarma (page 156), and it's filled with great sources of vitamins, fiber, and greens.

Makes 4 servings

4 cups Roasted Cauliflower Rice (page 140)

½ cup dried apricots, finely chopped

½ cup dried cranberries, finely chopped

½ cup parsley leaves, finely chopped

1 tablespoon lemon juice, plus more to serve

salt and pepper, to taste

yogurt, to serve

1. Combine the rice with the apricots, cranberries, and parsley.

2. Add the lemon juice, and salt and pepper, and mix well.

3. Serve with lemon, yogurt, and a savory protein dish.

Nutrition per serving: *200 calories, 4 g fat, 42 g carbohydrate, 14 g fiber, 9 g protein*

Tips

◆ I use Turkish unsulphured dried apricots, which are a bit darker than usual. For the cranberries, I use dried cranberries with no added sugar, sweetened with apple juice, and some sunflower oil added.

Creamed Spinach (Dairy-Free)

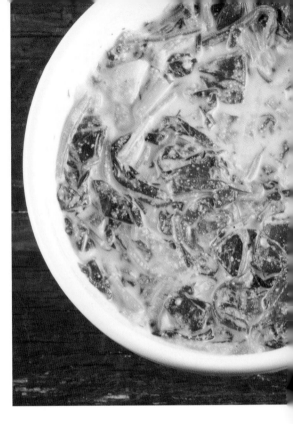

This healthy, dairy-free version of creamed spinach is fairly easy to prepare quickly. Soaking the cashews takes up most of the time, which you can bypass by making cashew cream ahead of time (refrigerate for about a week and use as needed).

Makes 4 servings

  1 cup raw cashews

  1 cup hot water, plus extra for soaking

  1 teaspoon lemon juice

  1½ teaspoons salt

  ¼ teaspoon ground nutmeg (optional)

  3 to 4 bunches of spinach, or about 32 ounces

  2 tablespoons olive oil

  1 cup chopped onion (red or yellow)

  4 cloves garlic, minced

1. Place the cashews in a bowl and cover with hot water. Soak them for 20 minutes or so then drain.

2. Add the soaked cashews, 1 cup of hot water, lemon juice, salt, and nutmeg, if using, to the blender and blend on high for about 1 minute, or until creamy and smooth. Set aside.

3. Chop the spinach in bite-size pieces and set aside.

4. Heat a large saucepan over medium heat. Add the olive oil and onion, and sauté for a few minutes or until they begin to soften.

5. Add the garlic and sauté for another minute.

6. Add the spinach and stir occasionally for a few minutes or until the spinach is wilted.

7. Turn off the heat and blend in about 1 cup of cashew cream.

8. Serve hot or warm. Store leftovers in the refrigerator for a few days.

Nutrition per serving: *275 calories, 19 g fat, 20 g carbohydrate, 3 g fiber, 8 g protein*

Zucchini Rollatini

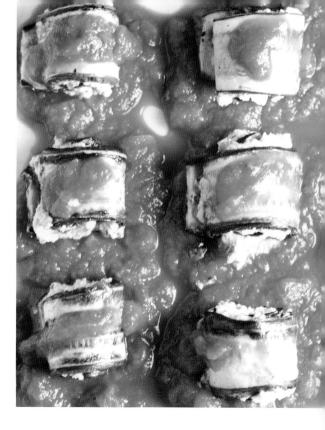

If it's hot outside you can bake these in your grill. Store them in the refrigerator for a few days and reheat at the same baking temperature.

Makes 24 rollatinis

4 large zucchini (as straight as possible, ends trimmed)

1 tablespoon olive oil

1 tablespoon salt

1 cup Ricotta Cheese (page 25)

handful spinach leaves, finely chopped

handful fresh basil leaves, finely chopped

2 cups Tomato Sauce (page 35)

1. Preheat the oven to 400°F/200 C°.

2. Using a mandolin or a knife, slice each zucchini into ¼ inch slices. You'll yield about 4 to 6 slices per zucchini, or up to 24 slices.

3. Lightly brush both sides with olive oil and sprinkle the salt on each side.

4. Grill or pan-fry the zucchini slices, about a minute on each side. They should be just soft enough to roll—don't let them get too soft or mushy.

5. In a medium bowl, add the cashew ricotta, spinach, and basil. Mix with a spoon or spatula to combine.

6. Spread about 1 tablespoon of the ricotta cheese mixture on each zucchini slice and then roll the slice up. Repeat for each zucchini slice.

7. Place the rolled zucchinis in a baking dish, pour the tomato sauce on top, and bake for about 15 minutes.

8. Cool for a few minutes then serve.

Nutrition per rollatini: *45 calories, 3 g fat, 4 g carbohydrate, 1 g fiber, 1 g protein*

Poultry, Meat, and Seafood

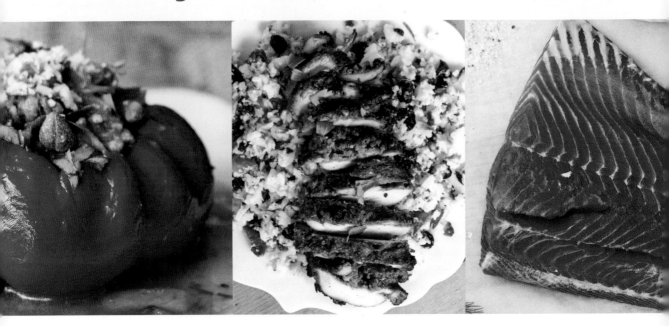

Here's a collection of recipes that are simple and flavorful versions of comfort food for meat and seafood lovers. Roasted or slow-cooked rotisserie chickens are the most requested birthday meals every year by my son, so you can imagine that I've mastered the art of grilling, roasting, and slow-cooking chicken. The other meal that never goes to waste is meatballs. These comfort meals will leave you with leftovers for lunch or dinner the next day or beyond. Or you can freeze half of a meal for a later date.

Falling-off-the-Bone Chicken

If you have a slow cooker, you'll love this recipe. If you don't have a slow cooker, I highly recommend saving up for one, because you can use it to make just about any warm meal, given enough time. To slow-cook chicken, just apply a healthy amount of dry rub to the skin and let it cook for several hours. That's all there is to it.

Makes 6 servings

4 carrots, peeled and trimmed

1 chicken (about 4 pounds), rinsed and patted dry

dry rub (1 teaspoon each garlic powder, mustard powder, salt, and paprika)

1 lemon, cut in half

2 garlic cloves, diced

1. Place the carrots on the bottom of the slow cooker.

2. Rub the chicken skin with the dry rub. Place the lemon and garlic inside the chicken cavity and set the chicken on top of the carrots in the cooker.

3. Cover and cook on a slow setting for 8 to 10 hours, or on a higher setting for 4 to 6 hours. The chicken is cooked when the juice coming out of a slice near a leg is clear and the leg moves easily or falls off at the joint.

4. If you want to brown the skin, heat your oven on broil (425°F/220°C), transfer the chicken to a broiling pan or a baking sheet, and set it in the oven for about 10 minutes.

5. Let the chicken cool for a few minutes and then slice. Store leftovers in the refrigerator, covered, for up to a few days, and consider making chicken broth out of the remains (see page 28).

Nutrition per serving: *425 calories, 8 g fat, 10 g carbohydrate, 2 g fiber, 89 g protein*

Classic Roasted Chicken

I can think of many ways to roast a chicken, and I've tried lots of them, but the simplest is often the best. This simple roasted chicken stays moist on the inside and crunchy on the outside. Gather some herbs, salt, and a lemon, and you have the makings of the most important component of a comforting meal. Plus, you can use the leftovers for Chicken Broth (page 28) or the Cherry Chicken Salad on page 59.

Often I'll make a chicken on Sunday night, then add the carcass and giblets to my slow cooker to make chicken broth for soups and other meals later in the week. When you're cooking for a crowd, I suggest roasting two chickens—if your oven can handle it—rather than buying a very large one. The larger your chicken, the longer it will take to roast and the drier the outside pieces will be. Also, with a pair of chickens you'll have more legs and wings to go around.

My favorite roasting setup for chicken is a rimmed baking sheet lined with parchment paper. I have a roasting rack that fits on the baking sheet, and then the chicken rests on the rack. The cleanup is a snap, and the drippings are easy to scoop up off the parchment paper to use for gravy. If you're finding that your chicken is becoming too dry on the outside about halfway through roasting, lower the temperature to about 325°F/165°C and roast it a bit longer than normal.

Makes 6 servings

1 roasting chicken (4 to 6 pounds; free-range if possible)

1 large lemon, sliced in half or quarters

2 large garlic cloves, sliced

1 tablespoon fresh thyme sprigs (or 1 teaspoon dried thyme)

1 tablespoon fresh or dried rosemary

2 tablespoons unsalted butter, melted

½ teaspoon salt, divided

1. Preheat your oven to 425°F/220°C.

2. Gently pull any excess fat off the chicken. Remove any parts from inside the cavity and then briefly rinse the chicken with water and pat dry with a paper towel. Drying off the skin ensures that it will be crunchy at the end of roasting and that the seasonings will stay put.

3. Set the chicken in a roasting rack. Place the lemon, garlic, and half the thyme and rosemary inside the chicken.

4. Gently lift the skin near the neck area and evenly spread ¼ teaspoon of salt under the skin. Rub the melted butter all over the outside of the chicken. Sprinkle the outside with the remaining ¼ teaspoon salt. Place the remaining thyme and rosemary between the legs and wings, as well as pressing some onto the body of the chicken.

5. Use string to tie the wings and legs close to the body. This is referred to as trussing a chicken, and I don't worry too much about the technique (although you can probably see many videos of this on the Internet). I just wrap the string around the body until all the parts are secure.

6. Roast the chicken for about an hour; test it by making a small cut inside a thigh to see if the juice from the chicken is clear. If it's still red, the chicken needs more time in the oven. If it's getting too dark on the outside, lightly rest some foil on top of the chicken.

Nutrition per serving: *434 calories, 12 g fat, 4 g carbohydrate, 0 g fiber, 88 g protein*

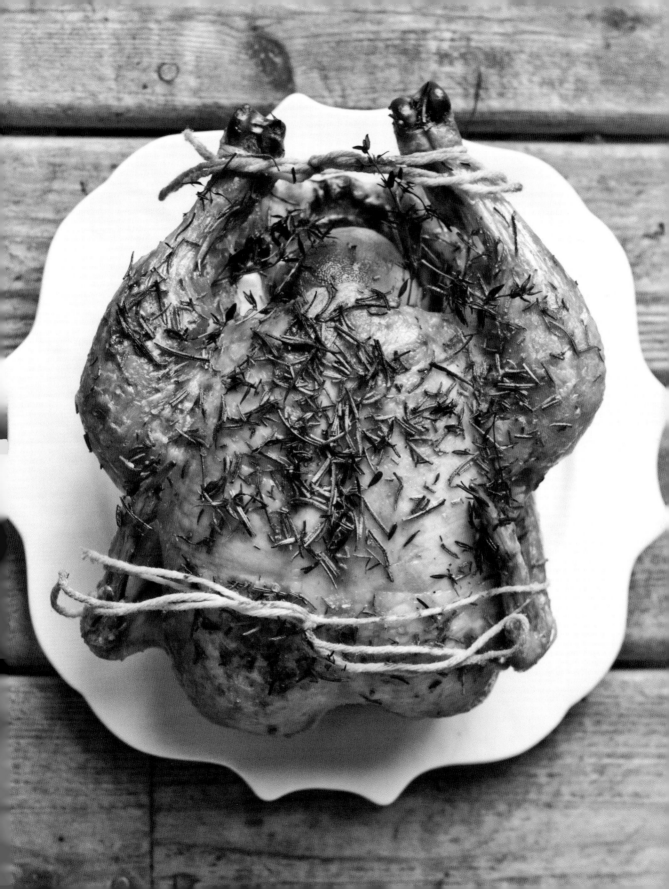

Chicken Tenders

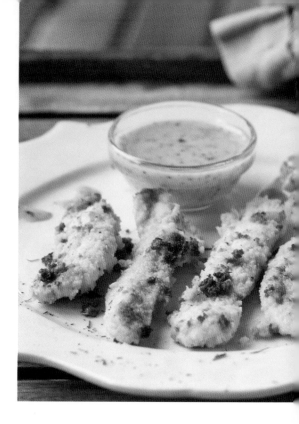

I've been making these chicken tenders for many years, but it wasn't until we started changing our diet that I began dredging them in almond flour. Now this is one of our most-loved recipes. It can be turned into chicken Parmesan, made into chicken sandwiches, chopped up and added to a salad, served over Zucchini Noodles (page 122), or just enjoyed as tenders to dip in a favorite sauce or dressing. Simple Ketchup (page 80) and Honey Mustard Dressing (page 79) are my family's favorites.

I've always used dill with this recipe, because the recipe started out as lemon-flavored tenders, with lemon juice dripped over them as they came out of the pan. If you don't have dill, you can do without it or use dried oregano, parsley, or basil instead.

Makes 4 servings

2 to 3 tablespoons olive oil or other cooking oil

1 to 1½ pounds chicken breast meat, sliced into pieces 1 to 2 inches long

1 egg, lightly beaten

1 tablespoon mustard (Dijon or stoneground works well)

1 cup blanched almond flour

¼ teaspoon salt, or to taste

¼ teaspoon dried dill weed

1. Heat the oil in a wide skillet over medium heat.

2. In a large bowl, stir together the chicken pieces, egg, and mustard until well blended.

3. In a separate bowl or on a plate, use a fork to stir together the almond flour, salt, and dill.

4. Dredge each piece of chicken in the flour mixture to fully coat it and then transfer it straight into the hot oil.

5. Fry the chicken pieces for 5 minutes or so on each side. Transfer to a plate and serve along with your favorite dip or dressing.

Nutrition per serving: *354 calories, 13 g fat, 2 g carbohydrate, 1 g fiber, 54 g protein*

Jamaican Jerk Chicken

This recipe is essentially finger food, and it's great for game nights, parties, and family gatherings.

Makes 6 servings

2 cups finely chopped scallions

1½ teaspoons dried thyme

2 cloves garlic, chopped

⅛ teaspoon cayenne pepper (optional)

2 teaspoons ground allspice

2 teaspoons ground dry mustard

1 teaspoon cinnamon

1 teaspoon salt

2 tablespoons lime juice

2 tablespoons honey

4 pounds skin-on chicken drumettes

1. In a large bowl, add all the ingredients except the chicken and stir to combine.

2. Add the chicken pieces and stir to coat with the marinade. Refrigerate for several hours, or overnight.

3. Preheat the oven to 400°F/200°C.

4. Prepare a baking sheet with parchment paper or a nonstick baking mat.

5. Place the chicken on the baking sheet and bake for 15 minutes.

6. Increase the oven temperature to 500°F/260°C and bake for another 5 to 10 minutes or until the chicken pieces are slightly blackened.

Nutrition per serving: *426 calories, 23 g fact, 9 g carbohydrate, 1 g fiber, 29 g protein*

Tips

- Drumettes are the thicker half of a chicken wing and resemble a small chicken leg. You can buy a large pack of wings and separate the drumette from the wingette and tip (ask the butcher to do it or do it yourself). You can also just bake the entire wing and then break them apart after they're cooked.

- You can omit the cayenne pepper if you're cooking for kids or those with milder tastes.

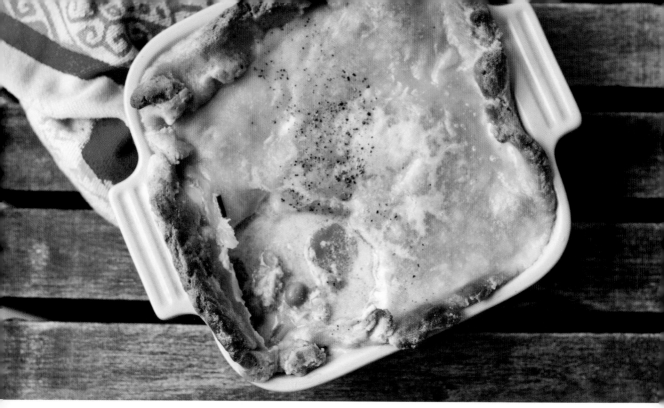

Chicken Pot Pie

I usually make pot pie when I have leftover roast chicken. You can use any kind of cooked chicken, though, leftover or not. A word about the egg wash: I love to add egg wash to crusts, when I remember to do so. If you can take the extra time, it will give the crust a very appealing patina.

You can bake this recipe a number of ways, depending on what you have on hand and how many will be partaking: 4 ramekins (about 6-ounce capacity); 1 (8-inch) round or square baking dish; 2 (6-inch) square baking dishes; or some variation of these dishes.

Makes 4 servings

2 cups shredded cooked chicken

2 cups Chicken Broth (page 28) or water

2 large carrots, peeled and sliced into coins

2 large celery stalks, sliced

1 cup peas (fresh or frozen)

½ teaspoon dried thyme, or ½ tablespoon fresh

¼ teaspoon sea salt, or to taste

¼ cup almond milk or other dairy-free milk, or SCD Yogurt (page 20; optional, for a creamy taste)

1 Butter Biscuits dough ball (page 101)

1 egg, beaten, for egg wash (optional)

1. Preheat your oven to 350°F/175°C.

2. Place the chicken, broth, carrots, celery, peas, thyme, salt, and milk or yogurt (if using) in a saucepan over low to medium heat and simmer for about 15 minutes, or until the carrots are tender.

3. Prepare the biscuit dough and chill in the freezer for 5 minutes.

4. Place the chilled dough between 2 sheets of parchment paper (or other nonstick material) and roll large enough to cover your baking dish or dishes.

5. Pour the chicken mixture into the baking dish (or dishes) about ¾ of the way full, leaving chunks of meat and veggies on top for the crust to rest on (avoid resting the crust on liquid, so it won't get soggy).

6. Rest the biscuit topping over the chicken mixture. Lightly brush the topping with egg wash, if you wish. Use a fork to make a few small punctures in the crust.

7. Bake for 15 minutes or so, depending on the size of your baking dish, or when the biscuit topping is beginning to brown and the filling is lightly bubbling. Let cool briefly and serve.

8. Refrigerate any leftovers, covered, for up to a few days. Reheat at 325°F/165°C for about 10 minutes or so, or until the filling is lightly bubbling.

Nutrition per serving: *400 calories, 12 g fat, 18 g carbohydrate, 10 g fiber, 28 g protein*

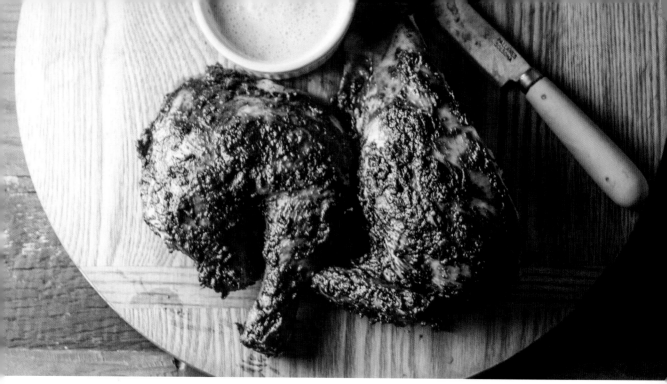

Peri Peri Chicken

This tangy chicken has a barbecue flavor without having to fire up a grill. And, while it's roasting, you can prepare a dipping sauce, such as Ranch Dressing (page 83) or Tzatziki (page 55). I recommend serving it with Jeweled Cauliflower Rice (page 143), No-Corn Cornbread (page 106), fresh greens, and steamed vegetables.

You can use a small, whole chicken, or chicken parts. If you use a whole chicken, you'll want to butterfly so you can spread the marinade on both sides and allow it to roast more quickly and evenly.

Makes 4 servings

1 large dried ancho chile

1 (4-pound) whole chicken or equivalent in chicken pieces

2 tablespoons smoked paprika

4 cloves garlic

1 tablespoon salt

¼ cup red wine vinegar

¼ cup olive oil

1. Soak the ancho chile in hot water for 10 minutes, or until soft.

2. Preheat the oven to 425°F/220°C.

3. Prepare a baking sheet with parchment paper or nonstick baking mat.

4. Butterfly the whole chicken (see instructions below).

5. Place the chicken on the baking sheet with the skin side down.

6. Remove the stem from the ancho chile. Add the ancho chile, paprika, garlic, salt, red wine vinegar, and olive oil to a food processor or blender, and process until it forms a thick paste.

7. Brush about ⅓ of the marinade on the chicken.

8. Place the chicken in the oven and bake for 15 minutes. Turn the chicken over, spread the remaining marinade over the chicken, and bake for another 30 minutes or until the chicken is fully cooked (the total baking time will depend on the size of your chicken).

9. Let the chicken rest for a few minutes and then slice it into parts.

10. Store leftovers in the refrigerator for a few days.

Nutrition per serving: *572 calories, 26 g fat, 7 g carbohydrate, 1 g fiber, 29 g protein*

Tips

◆ You can substitute 2 tablespoons of chili powder for the ancho chile.

◆ Lemon juice can be subbed for red wine vinegar.

◆ You can marinate the chicken overnight for a more flavorful result.

◆ How to butterfly a chicken: Rinse the chicken inside and out and remove the giblets, if they were included. Pat dry and place on a cutting board. Use kitchen scissors to cut along the spine on each side until you can remove it. Discard the spine and place the chicken skin up on a cutting board. Press down on the breast with the palms of your hands to flatten the chicken.

Chicken Shawarma

Grilled or baked, this chicken comes out equally flavorful. It's loaded with healthy spices, including my favorite, turmeric. For a milder, less spicy version, leave out the coriander and ginger.

Makes 6 servings

8 cloves garlic, minced

2 tablespoons ground cumin

2 tablespoons ground coriander

2 teaspoons ground turmeric

1 teaspoon ground ginger

2 teaspoons ground allspice

1½ teaspoons salt

¼ cup oil

2½ pounds skinless, boneless chicken thighs

1. Preheat the oven to the low broil setting.

2. Place the garlic, cumin, coriander, turmeric, ginger, allspice, salt, and oil in a food processor and pulse until it forms a paste.

3. Trim the chicken of excess fat and coat it completely with the spice paste.

4. Broil the chicken for 4 to 6 minutes on each side.

5. Serve hot. Store leftovers in the refrigerator for a few days or the freezer for a few months.

Nutrition per serving: *434 calories, 33 g fact, 13 g carbohydrate, 4 g fiber, 27 g protein*

Tips

◆ You can grill or broil this chicken.

◆ This recipe goes great with Jeweled Cauliflower Rice (page 143) or any of the other cauliflower rice recipes.

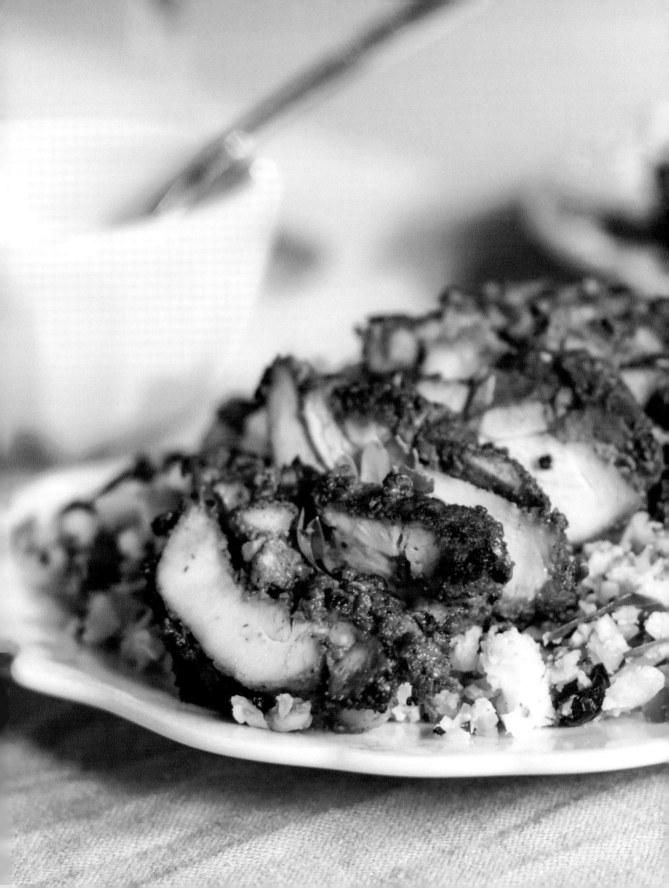

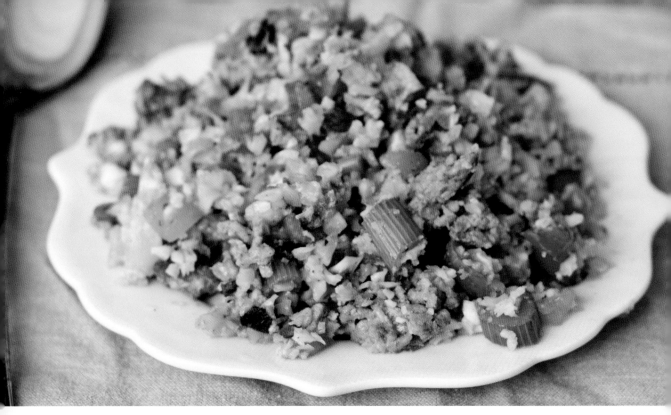

Dirty Rice

This one-dish meal is easy to reheat, so I usually make extra. Consider this recipe a somewhat loose description of dirty rice, because you can substitute a number of ingredients depending on what you have on hand or what you prefer. It also happens to go well with a side of salsa or gazpacho.

I always use Roasted Cauliflower Rice, but you can mix and match the protein sources as you prefer. While I happen to like chicken liver, many don't, so I avoid using it in large amounts. Everyone loves bacon, so I always include that. If you don't use bacon, you'll want to add a bit more salt, since the bacon contributes quite a bit of saltiness.

Makes 4 servings

½ cup chicken livers (optional; I only use them from guaranteed healthy, free-range chickens)

1 teaspoon cooking oil (if using chicken livers)

4 slices bacon, chopped into small pieces

½ pound ground pork (or other ground meat)

½ cup finely diced onion

4 small celery stalks, finely diced

½ cup finely chopped green or red bell pepper

½ cup Chicken Broth (page 28), Vegetable Broth page 31, or water

½ teaspoon garlic powder

½ teaspoon paprika

pinch of cayenne pepper (optional, for a bit of heat)

recipe for Roasted Cauliflower Rice (page 140)

sea salt and pepper, to taste

1. If you're using the chicken livers, place them in a warmed skillet over medium heat with 1 teaspoon cooking oil, and cook, stirring occasionally. When they are browned and no longer red on the outside, remove them from the pan. Dice them finely, and set aside.

2. Add the bacon pieces to the same skillet and cook over medium heat until crispy on the edges, about 5 minutes. Leave the bacon fat in the skillet for the next step.

3. Spread the ground pork across the surface of the skillet and brown it for about 5 minutes over high heat without stirring.

4. Once the pork is browned on the bottom, break it up into small pieces and lower the heat back to medium.

5. Add the onion, celery, and bell pepper and cook for another 5 minutes, stirring occasionally. Cook until the onions start to become translucent.

6. Add the chicken broth, garlic powder, paprika, and cayenne pepper (if using) to the skillet. Cook, stirring occasionally, until the stock has boiled off.

7. Add the cauliflower rice to the skillet along with the chicken livers, if using; stir to blend well. Add salt and pepper to taste.

8. Remove from the heat and serve warm. You can store leftovers in the refrigerator, covered, for up to a few days.

Nutrition per serving: *331 calories, 21 g fat, 10 g carbohydrate, 3 g fiber, 25 g protein*

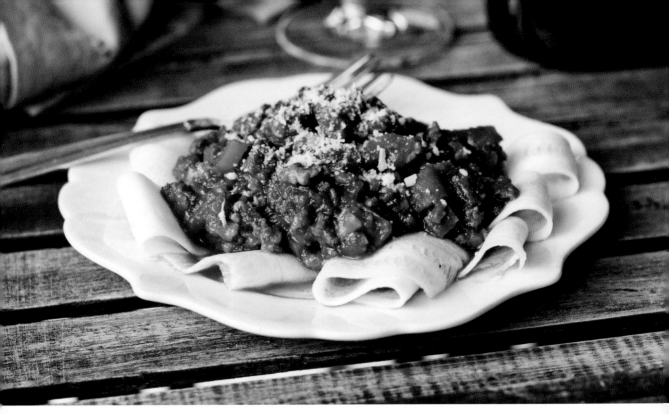

Ragu Bolognese (Red Meat Sauce)

This is a classic recipe for red meat sauce that I've simplified a bit and made dairy-free. I tend to use ground beef and pork, but you can use sausage meat or substitute something else. It's delicious over Focaccia (page 119), Squash Ribbon Noodles (page 126), or Garlic Toasts (page 120).

Makes 8 servings

4 tablespoons olive oil, divided

1 pound ground pork

1 pound ground beef

½ cup finely diced onion

½ cup finely diced carrots

¼ cup finely chopped celery

1 tablespoon fresh thyme, or 1 teaspoon dried thyme

3 medium garlic cloves, minced

2 tablespoons Tomato Paste (page 35)

½ cup dry red wine

4 ounces pancetta, finely diced (ham or bacon also work)

1 (28-ounce) can crushed tomatoes

3 cups beef broth (or chicken or vegetable broth, or water)

1. Heat 1 tablespoon olive oil in a skillet over medium heat. Add the pork and beef, breaking it up with a spatula. Brown for a few minutes, and then remove the browned meat from the pan and set aside in a large saucepan you'll use for cooking the ragu.

2. Add the onions, carrots, and celery to the skillet and cook for about 5 minutes, stirring occasionally. Add the thyme, garlic, and tomato paste and cook for another minute or so.

3. Pour the wine into the pan and cook for another few minutes, or until the wine is reduced by half.

4. Pour the frying pan mixture into a large saucepan along with the meat and all the remaining ingredients, stirring to combine well. Simmer for about 45 minutes on a low heat lightly covered, or until the sauce is thick but easily stirred. About halfway through cooking remove the cover and if the sauce is not thick enough, let some of the moisture evaporate. If it is too thick, add some water and cook for a few more minutes.

5. Serve warm; or let cool, cover, and store in the refrigerator for several days or in the freezer for a few months.

Nutrition per serving: *425 calories, 28 g fat, 7 g carbohydrate, 1 g fiber, 30 g protein*

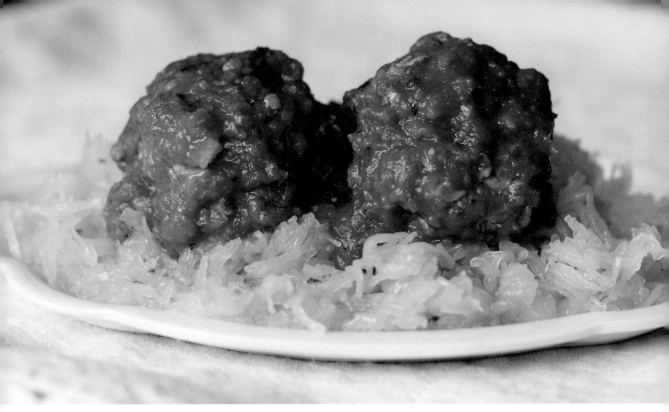

Fennel Pesto Meatballs

I use pesto for many kinds of recipes—it's a terrific way to pack greens and flavor into a dish, and it's so easy to make. I've been known to eat just pesto on toast, or with scrambled eggs. In this case, the pesto is part of the meatball recipe, and I use whatever fresh greens I have on hand. It could be kale, parsley, basil, or arugula. It's nice to change it up to give the meatballs a different flavor, or depending on the ground meat and sauce base you're using. If you're not eating eggs, no worries. These meatballs will stay together without the egg.

Makes 10 (2-meatball) servings

½ cup grated Parmesan cheese

½ cup fresh parsley (or other greens, such as basil, kale, or arugula)

½ tablespoon fennel seeds

1 medium garlic clove

½ teaspoon salt

1 pound ground meat (beef and pork, or turkey and chicken)

1 egg

1 tablespoon ghee (page 23) or high-heat oil

2 cups Classic Marinara Sauce (page 78) or a trustworthy jar of sauce (see Product Sources, page 214)

1. Combine the Parmesan, parsley, fennel seeds, garlic, and salt in the bowl of a food processor and process until finely ground, like pesto.

2. Place the pesto, meat, and egg in a bowl and combine gently, using a spatula or fork.

3. Melt the ghee or oil over medium heat in a large Dutch oven or saucepan (one that has a cover).

4. Using an ice cream scoop or spoon, shape the meat mixture into meatballs and place in the hot skillet, leaving space between the meatballs.

5. Brown the meatballs briefly on all sides so that they hold together. Transfer them to a plate and set aside. Drain the excess fat from the pan.

6. Pour the marinara sauce into the pan and return the meatballs to the pan as well. Cover and bring the sauce to a steady simmer. Reduce the heat and simmer for 10 minutes or so and then serve; or let cool, cover, and refrigerate for a few days, or freeze for later use.

Nutrition per serving: *197 calories, 12 g fat, 3 g carbohydrate, 1 g fiber, 18 g protein*

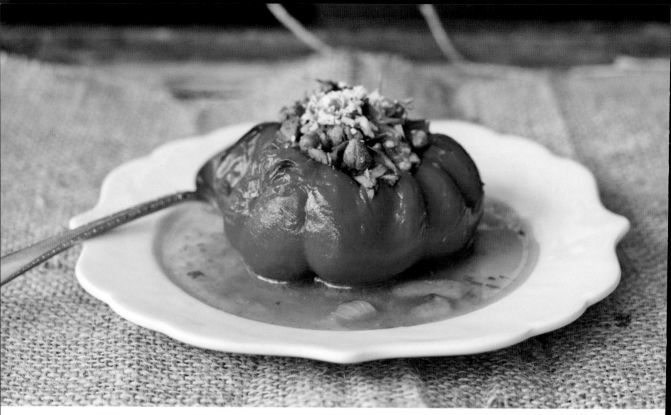

Stuffed Bell Peppers

I have a personal affection for bell peppers, especially the red and orange versions, which I think stems from the fact that they are the sweetest. The red pepper happens to offer the most vitamins and nutrients, evident in its color. Pair that with a savory filling, and you have a compact meal elegantly held together in a vitamin-rich fruit (yes, it's actually a fruit, because it has seeds).

Makes 8 servings

8 medium red bell peppers (or yellow, orange, or green)

1 tablespoon olive oil, plus more for coating the peppers

1 small onion, diced into small pieces

1 pound ground meat (chicken, beef, or turkey)

4 cups Classic Marinara Sauce (page 78) or other tomato sauce, divided

2 tablespoons capers

¼ cup finely chopped fresh parsley

½ cup grated Parmesan cheese (or other aged hard cheese)

1. Preheat your oven to 350°F / 175°C.

2. Cut the stem tops off the peppers and take out the seeds.

3. Steam or boil the peppers in a pot of lightly salted water for about 8 minutes, or until they are slightly soft and brighter in color. Drain and set aside.

4. Place 1 tablespoon of olive oil and the onions in a skillet over medium heat and cook for about 5 minutes, or until they start to turn translucent.

5. Add the meat and cook for another 5 minutes, stirring occasionally. Turn off the heat and stir in 1 cup of the marinara sauce, the capers, parsley, and the cheese. Stir occasionally, breaking up the meat with a spatula.

6. Lightly coat each pepper inside and outside with olive oil, then spoon the meat filling into the peppers.

7. Pour 1 cup of marinara sauce into a shallow baking dish about 9 x 11 inches in size, adding water as necessary to cover the bottom of the dish. Set the stuffed peppers in the baking dish and bake for about 12 minutes.

8. Serve the remaining marinara sauce with the peppers.

> **Nutrition per serving:** *293 calories, 16 g fat, 13 g carbohydrate, 4 g fiber, 23 g protein*

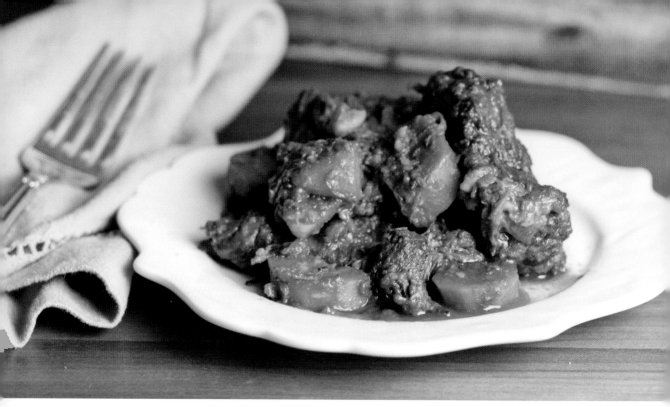

Braised Short Ribs and Carrots

You can make this slow-cooking meal in a slow cooker or in a Dutch oven or heavy saucepan on your stovetop. It can keep going until you're ready for it, and it can tolerate other root vegetable additions (added about 1 hour before it's done) as well as last-minute additions such as peas and diced zucchini (added 15 minutes before it's done). At around 4 hours, it's usually done, but another hour or so and the meat will fall off the bone and melt in your mouth. The cut of meat means this does produce a lot of fat that floats to the top, so I always skim the fat off the top after letting it cool for a bit.

Makes 4 servings

1 tablespoon ghee (page 23) or cooking oil

4 pounds beef short ribs (grass-fed, if possible)

simple rub (equal amounts garlic powder, onion powder, mustard powder, and salt)

1 cup chopped onion (about 1 small onion)

4 cloves garlic, chopped

1 cup broth (beef, chicken, or vegetable) or water

½ teaspoon salt

1 tablespoon honey

¾ cup (6 ounces) Tomato Paste (page 35)

¼ cup chopped fresh parsley

4 carrots, peeled and chopped

1. Heat the ghee or oil in a large skillet over medium heat. Coat each rib with the rub and then lightly brown on all sides in the skillet. Set aside.

2. In a slow cooker or a Dutch oven or large saucepan, place the onion and garlic on the bottom and then add the broth, salt, honey, and tomato paste. Stir to combine.

3. Place the ribs on top of the onion mixture and cover the slow cooker or pan.

4. Set the slow cooker to high or the stovetop burner between low and medium. Cover and cook for 4 hours and then add the parsley and carrots to the mixture; cover again and continue cooking.

5. After 5 to 6 hours of cooking, the meat should be falling off the bone and the carrots should be quite tender. Turn off the slow cooker or remove the pan from the burner, cool for a few minutes, and skim the fat off the top.

6. Serve warm; or cover and store in the refrigerator for a few days or in the freezer for up to about a month.

Nutrition per serving: *221 calories, 10 g fat, 23 g carbohydrate, 4 g fiber, 18 g protein*

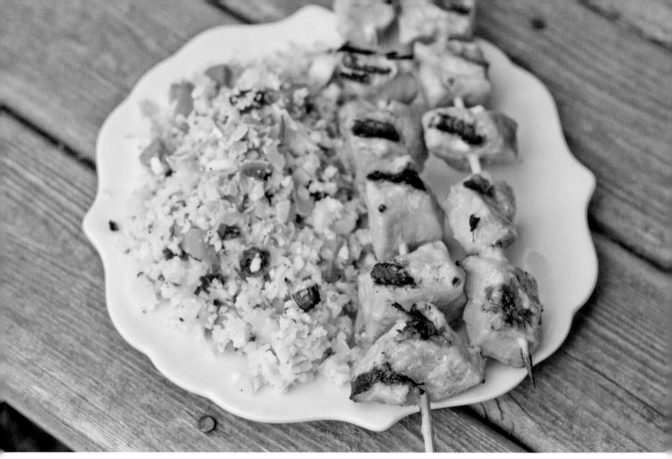

Citrus Tuna Kebabs

Seafood and citrus go especially well together, and I love the balance of sweet, salty, and citrus in this dish. It cooks quickly, so I suggest preparing everything ahead of time and then chilling it until you're ready to grill and serve. Serve these kebobs with Orange Cauliflower Couscous (page 138).

I'd estimate that I have tuna only a few times a year, and when I do, I buy only sustainable tuna. If you don't have access to tuna, you can substitute halibut or another fish that cooks well in cubed cuts.

Makes 6 servings

2 pounds filleted ahi tuna (troll or pole-caught is best)

¼ cup olive oil

2 tablespoons grated fresh ginger

1 tablespoon grated orange zest

¼ cup fresh orange juice

¼ cup honey

1 or 2 pinches of sea salt

1. Cut the tuna into bite-size cubes.

2. Blend the tuna cubes with all the other ingredients in a glass bowl. Cover and let marinate in the refrigerator for at least 30 minutes.

3. Thread the tuna onto skewers.

4. Preheat a grill to medium heat, and grill the tuna kebobs for about 5 minutes on each side, for a total of 10 minutes on the grill. Watch them carefully because they tend to cook quickly.

> **Nutrition per serving:** *290 calories, 15 g fat, 13 g carbohydrate, 0 g fiber, 35 g protein*

Parties

Bring food that you know you can eat. There are great dishes that are party-safe, and you may be surprised when your dish is the first to go.

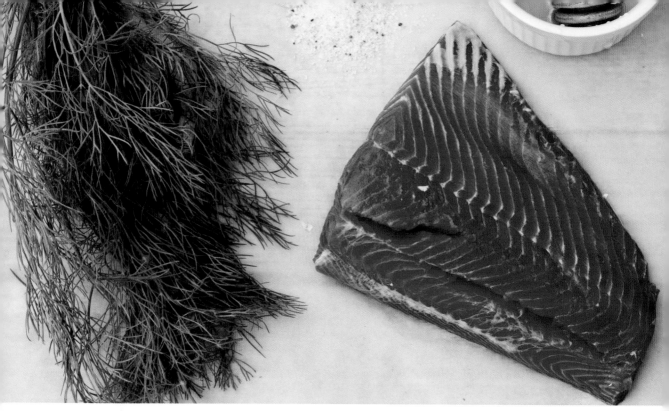

Cured Salmon (Gravlax)

Gravlax is salted salmon that has been cured for a few days—not to be confused with smoked salmon, which is drier and has a smoky flavor. While gravlax is easy to make, you'll need to plan ahead by at least a day. The reward will be worth the time. I prefer my salmon a bit less salty, so I tend to hold back a bit on the salt and only cure the fish for a day. It's up to you, though. If the salmon tastes too salty to you after curing, you can add some water and let it cure for a few more hours to let the water pull out the salt. The opposite will also work—if it's not salty enough, add salt and let it cure for a few more hours. And if it's not sweet enough, add honey and cure for a few more hours. You can substitute a citrus cure for the dill, using about 1 teaspoon grated lemon or lime zest on each side.

Try cured salmon in a crêpe (page 103) with capers and Herbed Cream Cheese (page 22), or mixed into scrambled eggs with a side of toasted Simple Sandwich Bread (page 92).

Makes 4 servings

2 pounds filleted salmon

¼ cup fresh chopped dill, divided

¼ cup honey, divided

¼ cup kosher sea salt (or other coarse salt)

1. Rinse the salmon and pat dry with a paper towel.

2. Place half the dill and half the honey in the bottom of a glass baking dish large enough to hold the salmon.

3. Coat both sides of the salmon with the salt, sprinkling it evenly.

4. Lay the salmon on top of the honey and dill in the baking dish. Cover with the remaining salt, honey, and dill.

5. Cover with plastic wrap and place a heavy plate or dish over the salmon. Refrigerate for 24 hours to cure.

6. When the salmon is fully cured, it will be darker and firmer. Drain off the liquid and rinse off the salt, honey, and dill; pat dry.

7. Slice thinly to serve—perhaps with Herbed Goat Cheese on toasted Simple Sandwich Bread. Store in a sealed container in the refrigerator for up to a week or so.

Nutrition per serving: *334 calories, 10 g fat, 17 g carbohydrate, 0 g fiber, 42 g protein*

Seek Out Sustainable Seafood

Fish are rich in healthy oils, protein, minerals, and vitamins. Unfortunately, many types are also endangered due to overfishing and toxicity in our waterways and oceans. An excellent way to determine if a fish is in season, local, safe, and sustainable is to use the Monterey Bay Aquarium's Seafood Watch website (montereybayaquarium.org). There's also a handy pocket guide you can carry in your wallet, and there's an app you can install on your phone to check while you're shopping.

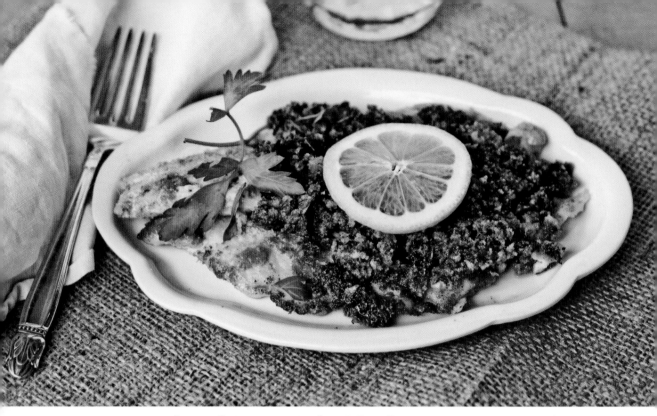

Pan-Fried White Fish (Sole Meuniere)

Here's a dish that's both easy and elegant. While the classic recipe calls for Dover sole, you can use any white fish, sliced somewhat thin. As for most fish dishes, I recommend preparing the ingredients ahead of time, since the sole cooks relatively quickly. You can keep it warm in the oven before serving.

This pairs well with Roasted Cauliflower Rice (page 140).

Makes 4 servings

½ cup blanched almond flour

¼ teaspoon sea salt

6 tablespoons unsalted butter or ghee (page 23), divided

6 Dover sole fillets (3 to 4 ounces each)

1 cup finely chopped fresh Italian parsley, plus more for garnish

3 lemons, both juice and zest (about ½ cup juice and 1½ tablespoons grated zest)

1 lemon, sliced for garnish

1. Blend the almond flour and salt on a plate, for dredging.

2. In a wide skillet over medium heat, melt 4 tablespoons of the butter or ghee. Keep cooking until it begins to bubble and turns slightly brown but isn't burnt. (Ghee won't turn brown, because the solids have been removed.)

3. While the butter is melting, dredge the fish fillets in the almond flour.

4. Place the fillets in the pan when the butter is starting to brown. Fry for about a minute on each side, then transfer to a warm plate or a baking dish in a warm oven.

5. Add the remaining 2 tablespoons butter or ghee to the skillet along with the 1 cup parsley, lemon juice and zest, and any almond flour remaining after dredging. Cook for about 1 minute.

6. Cover the fillets with the parsley-lemon sauce and serve garnished with the lemon slices.

Nutrition per serving: *331 calories, 21 g fat, 3 g carbohydrate, 1 g fiber, 33 g protein*

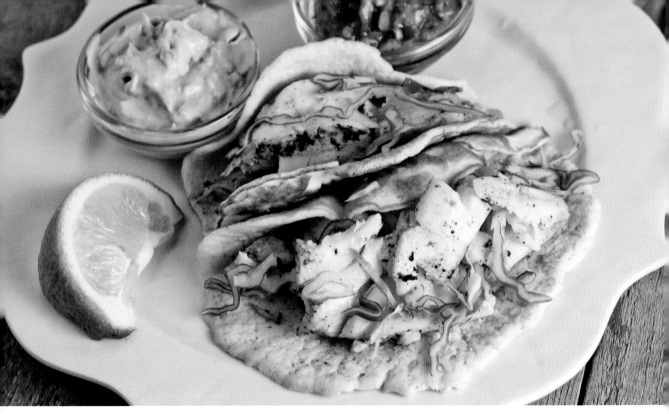

Fish Tacos

This is actually a combination of recipes from this book. And while you don't have to, it's nice to soak the fish in the lime juice for at least an hour before you plan to cook it.

Makes 4 tacos

about 1 pound white fish fillets (cod, halibut, or other)

1 lime, plus a few thinly sliced wedges

Avocado Crema (page 87)

Tortillas (page 118)

Creamy Coleslaw (page 59)

1 tablespoon unsalted butter

¼ teaspoon salt

pico de gallo (optional)

1. Soak the fish in the juice of 1 lime.

2. Prepare the Avocado Crema, tortillas, and coleslaw.

3. Place a large skillet over medium heat. Add the butter to the skillet and heat until it begins to turn light brown.

4. Add the fish fillets and cook for about 8 minutes, turning in between, or cook on each side until cooked through and lightly flaking.

5. Assemble the tacos and serve with lime wedges and pico de gallo.

Nutrition per taco: *310 calories, 32 g fat, 6 g carbohydrate, 4 g fiber, 28 g protein*

Parchment-Baked Fish

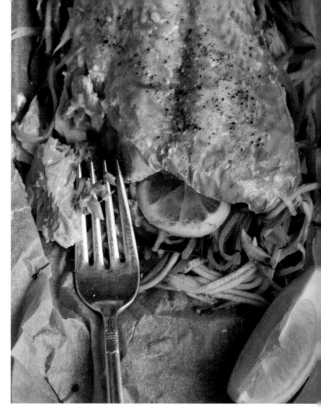

I love the simplicity and elegance of this meal. It's like a meal packet for one, and you can use any kind of fish, not only salmon. Just adjust the baking time according to the thickness of the fish.

The following amounts are for a single packet per person, so you'll want to double or quadruple them depending on how many you're serving. For four people, for example, you'll want two carrots, two zucchini, and two lemons.

This dish goes well with Roasted Cauliflower Rice (page 140).

Makes 1 serving

½ medium zucchini, thinly diced or julienned

½ medium carrot, peeled and thinly diced or julienned

1 shallot or ½ small onion, thinly sliced

1 tablespoon unsalted butter, ghee (page 23), or olive oil

2 or 3 thin lemon slices and 1 lemon wedge

¼ teaspoon dried dill weed or ½ tablespoon fresh dill (or other herb)

1 (6 to 8-ounce) salmon fillet

salt and pepper to taste

splash of dry white wine (about 1 tablespoon; optional)

1. Preheat your oven to 350°F/175°C.

2. Cut a piece of parchment paper about 12 x 14 inches. Arrange the zucchini, carrot, and onion slices in the middle of the paper.

3. Place the butter, lemon slices, and dill on top of the veggies.

4. Place the salmon fillet on top of the veggies, and sprinkle with salt and pepper. Optionally, pour about 1 tablespoon white wine over the fish.

5. Bring the longer sides of the parchment paper together, covering the salmon. Crimp the edges together, forming a sealed parchment packet, and place the sealed packet on a baking sheet.

6. Bake for 15 minutes, or until the salmon has some white on top and the veggies are bubbling.

7. Keep the packet closed until ready to eat. Serve with a lemon wedge to squeeze over the salmon.

Nutrition per serving: *359 calories, 16 g fat, 13 g carbohydrate, 4 g fiber, 43 g protein*

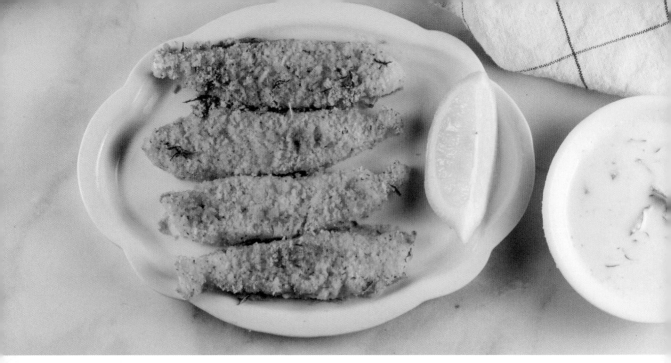

Fish Sticks

Fish sticks are a fun way to prepare coated, baked fish. I use thick-cut fish that holds together well when baked, such as halibut, tuna, cod, or salmon. You can fry this in a skillet as well; just preheat your skillet, follow the directions below, and then add the coated fish pieces.

Makes 4 servings

2 pounds halibut (or other firm fish)

1 cup almond flour

1 teaspoon dried dill

1 teaspoon sweet paprika

1 teaspoon salt

lemon, to serve

1. Preheat the oven to 400°F/200°C.

2. Prepare a baking sheet with parchment paper or a nonstick baking mat.

3. Slice the fish into strips, thick enough to prevent them from falling apart too easily.

4. Add the almond flour, dill, paprika, and salt to a medium bowl and blend well with a fork.

5. Dredge each fish slice in the flour mixture until all sides are coated, and place on the baking sheet.

6. Bake for 10 minutes, or until the fish is cooked through.

7. Serve with a squeeze of lemon or lemon slices, Simple Ketchup (page 80), or Tartar Sauce (page 89).

> **Nutrition per serving:** *293 calories, 9 g fat, 2 g carbohydrate, 1 g fiber, 48 g protein*

Sweet Treats

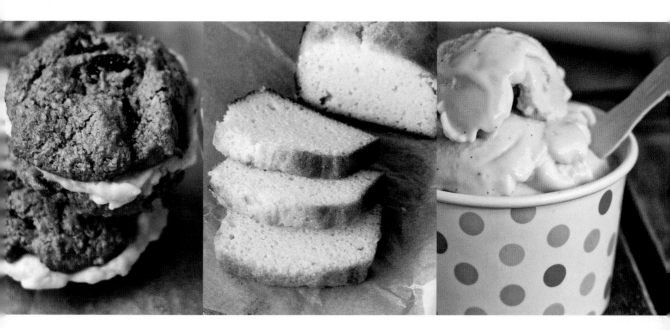

I've been an avid baker all my life. It started with chocolate chip cookies at about 9 years of age, and I've been going strong since then. I hadn't baked with almond or coconut flour until I stumbled upon SCD, but now I love using these nutritious and flavorful flours.

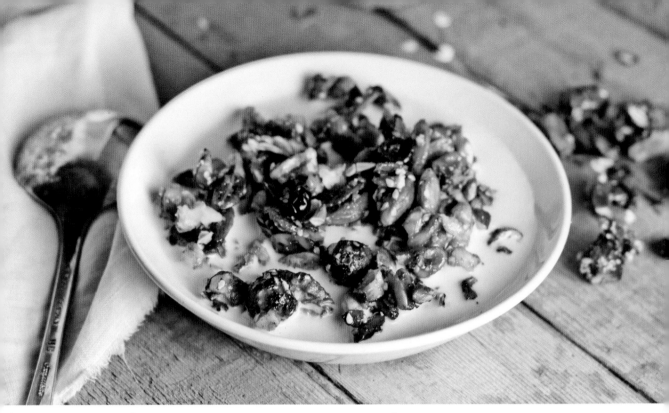

Crunchy No-Grain Granola

Granola is easy to make, and it's more affordable when you make it yourself. Here's a simple granola formula that I use, allowing me not to think too much about how much of how many things I'm adding. I just add 6 cups of my favorite stuff, plus a bit of salt, vanilla, and oil, and off it goes on a baking sheet to the oven.

You can also make this nut-free if you're avoiding nuts or feel you're eating too many nut-based goodies—which can be a hazard with all those wonderful almond flour baked goods. Add granola on top of yogurt or ice cream, or pour cold almond milk (or other dairy-free milk) over a bowl of it. And it's a highly portable protein/carbohydrate snack.

Leave the dried fruit out of the mix until the granola has finished baking. This prevents the dried fruit from becoming dry and hard. For a less chunky, finer-textured granola, chop up at least half of the larger nuts, such as the hazelnuts and almonds. I wrap them in a dishtowel and gently smash them with a hammer. To make the granola less sweet, reduce the honey to about ⅓ cup.

Makes 8 (¾-cup) servings

1 cup raw pecans

1 cup raw almonds

1 cup raw pumpkin seeds

1 cup raw walnuts

1 cup raw hazelnuts

¼ cup raw sesame seeds

1 tablespoon coconut oil, ghee (page 23), or unsalted butter, melted

½ teaspoon salt

¼ teaspoon ground cinnamon

½ cup honey

1 teaspoon vanilla extract

½ cup dried cherries (or raisins or dried cranberries)

1. Preheat your oven to 300°F/150°C. Line a rimmed baking sheet with parchment paper or a nonstick baking mat.

2. In a large bowl, combine all the ingredients except for the dried cherries, stirring until the nuts and seeds are well coated.

3. Spread the mixture evenly across the prepared baking sheet. Bake for 10 minutes, then use a spatula to shuffle the granola around so that it bakes evenly.

4. Bake for another 10 to 15 minutes, or until the granola begins to brown. The pieces should be slightly sticky to touch but not *too* sticky. Remove it from the oven, separating the pieces before they cool and clump together.

5. Let cool completely (for at least 20 minutes) and then mix in the dried fruit. Store the granola in a sealed container at room temperature for several weeks or in the refrigerator for a few months.

Nutrition per serving: *587 calories, 46 g fat, 38 g carbohydrate, 8 g fiber, 14 g protein*

Blondies

In case you're wondering, blondies are kind of like vanilla brownies. There's no flour used in this recipe—just almond butter. These are soft and chewy like you'd expect from a brownie. Read the tips if you'd like to create a more caramel-like flavor using this recipe.

Makes 16 squares

8 ounces unsalted almond butter	1 teaspoon vanilla extract
½ cup honey	½ teaspoon baking soda
1 large egg	½ teaspoon salt

1. Preheat the oven to 350°F/175°C.

2. Line an 8 x 8-inch baking pan with parchment paper or grease generously.

3. Add all the ingredients to a large bowl and blend well with a spoon.

4. Scoop the batter into the baking pan and distribute evenly with a spatula or spoon.

5. Bake for 25 minutes, or until a toothpick inserted in the center comes out mostly clean. It may rise a bit before it's done baking.

6. Cool and slice. Store covered in the refrigerator for a week or so, or freeze for a few months.

> **Nutrition per square:** *165 calories, 9 g fat, 21 g carbohydrate, 2 g fiber, 4 g protein*

Tips

- To make this into almond toffee brownies, add 2 tablespoons of freeze-dried coffee plus 2 tablespoons hot water in step 4.

- You can also add about ½ cup of dark coffee or a bit less of espresso.

- You can use any nut butter or seed butter for this recipe. For example, to make it nut-free, use pumpkin butter or sunflower seed butter. Also, feel free to use crunchy almond butter to get a more "toffee" texture to the recipe.

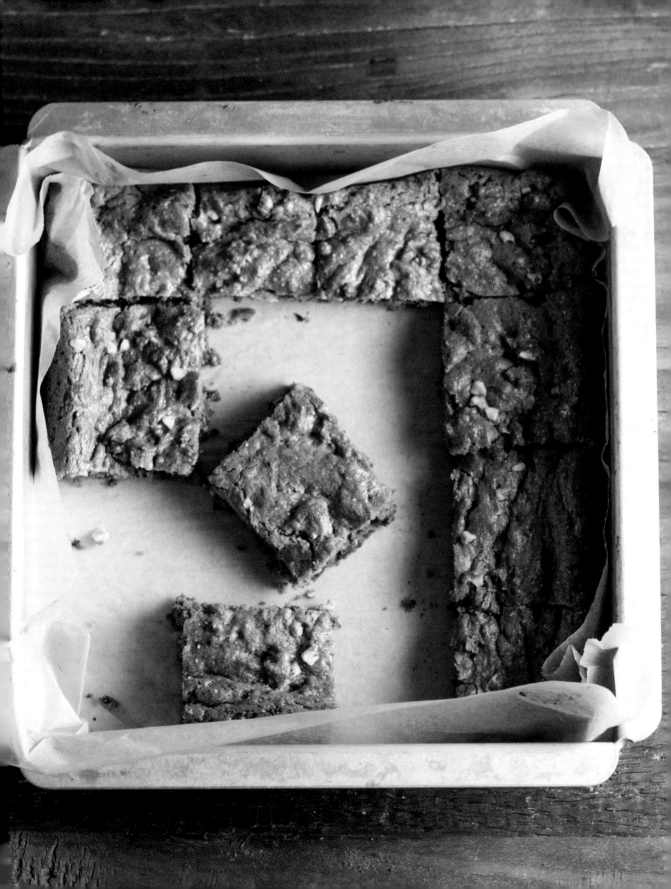

Strawberry Fruit Roll-Ups

Sweet and tart, fruit roll-ups, or fruit leather, are a fast snack and pick-me-up for kids of all ages. Use just about any kind of berry, although some may work better than others depending on the ripeness and sweetness of the fruit.

Generally, apple, apricots, berries with seeds, cherries, peaches, pears, and strawberries work well on their own as fruit leather. Blueberries and bananas are best combined with another fruit that works well on its own.

Makes 24 fruit rolls

> 2 pounds strawberries
>
> 2 tablespoons honey (or more depending on the sweetness of the fruit)

1. Add the strawberries and honey to a food processor or blender. Blend until it turns into a smooth, thick liquid.

2. If you want to remove seeds, now is the time to add the puree to a fine mesh strainer and press it through. Discard the seeds.

3. Spread the puree across the tray of a dehydrator.

4. Dehydrate for 8 to 10 hours at 105°F/40°C, or a bit higher if you prefer to speed up the process.

5. When the fruit layer is dry, peel it off the surface and eat. To store, place the leather on a piece of parchment or wax paper and roll it up to cover. Store sealed at room temperature for a few days, or in the refrigerator for a few weeks.

Nutrition per fruit roll: *6 calories, 0 g fat, 2 g carbohydrate, 0 g fiber, 0 g protein*

Tips

- To remove the seeds from fruit, press the mashed fruit through a fine mesh strainer. For this recipe, I used only strawberries and left the seeds in the puree.

- Frozen fruit works well in the recipe; you can freeze berries in season and make all year long.

- I use a dehydrator for this recipe, but if you don't have one, spread the puree in step 3 onto a nonstick baking mat and place in the oven for about 8 hours at 140°F/60°C.

- Instead of storing the full fruit whole, cut strips of it with scissors to store individual roll-ups.

Cinnamon Cookie

This is a quick and easy recipe for a chewy, buttery, cinnamon cookie. And it's egg-free, which is hard to come by in a grain-free cookie.

To make this dairy-free, substitute shortening or coconut oil for the butter.

Makes 20 cookies

2 cups blanched almond flour

1/8 teaspoon salt

1/4 teaspoon baking soda

1 teaspoon ground cinnamon

1/3 cup honey

4 tablespoons unsalted butter, melted

1. Preheat your oven to 275°F/135°C.

2. Prepare a baking sheet with parchment paper or a nonstick baking mat.

3. Combine the ingredients in a large mixing bowl and blend with a spoon.

4. With a spoon or your hands, create small balls of dough (about 1 tablespoon) and place them on the baking sheet.

5. Flatten each cookie ball with your palm or, if you prefer, flatten each cookie with a fork to create a pattern.

6. Bake for 20 minutes then turn the cookies over.

7. Lower the temperature to 175°F and bake for another 10 minutes.

8. Cool for 10 minutes or so.

> **Nutrition per cookie:** *102 calories, 8 g fat, 7 g carbohydrate, 1 g fiber, 2 g protein*

General Advice for Baking Success

Before you dive into a recipe, here are some tips to bring you baking success:

• Read the recipe at least twice (I even reread my familiar favorites every so often).

• Bring all your ingredients to room temperature, if possible. (I must admit I'm guilty of using cold ingredients. To counteract this, I bring the batter to room temperature before baking it.)

• Prepare baking pans and baking sheets at the beginning (makes life that much easier).

• Check on your baking goodies about 10 minutes before they're supposed to be done. Baking times are approximate and depend on a number of factors, including your oven, the altitude, any swapped ingredients, the pan you use, etc.

Ginger Snap Cookies

This is a sweet and spicy cookie with a snap.

Makes 20 cookies

2 cups blanched almond flour

¼ teaspoon salt

¼ teaspoon baking soda

1 teaspoon ground cinnamon

2 teaspoons ground ginger

½ teaspoon ground cloves

⅓ cup honey

4 tablespoons unsalted butter, melted

1. Preheat your oven to 350°F/175°C.

2. Prepare a baking sheet with parchment paper or a nonstick baking mat.

3. Add the flour, salt, baking soda, cinnamon, ginger, and cloves to a large bowl and blend well.

4. Add the honey and butter to the bowl and blend until a soft dough forms. If it's too soft, put it in the freezer for a few minutes.

5. Shape 1 tablespoon of dough into a ball and place it on the baking sheet. Repeat for the rest of the dough.

6. Press each cookie down with your hands or a fork.

7. Bake for 10 minutes or until they are golden brown.

8. Cool for a few minutes.

Nutrition per cookie: *54 calories, 4 g fat, 5 g carbohydrate, 0 g fiber, 1 g protein*

Tips

◆ If you store a rolled dough log in the freezer wrapped in parchment or wax paper, you can bake a batch of these at a moment's notice. Just preheat your oven and bake as directed.

Gingerbread Biscotti

Biscotti goes great with a cup of tea or coffee, a glass of dairy-free milk, or just by itself. While the recipe uses almond flour, the process is similar to the classic technique of double-baking the cookies.

Makes 30 biscotti

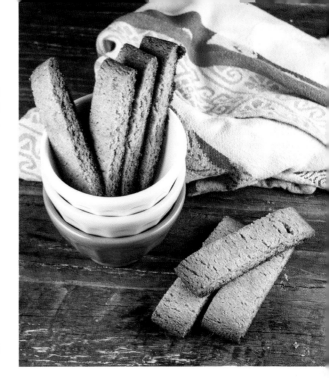

2 cups blanched almond flour

¼ teaspoon sea salt

¼ teaspoon baking soda

1 teaspoon ground cinnamon

2 teaspoons ground ginger

½ teaspoon ground cloves

⅓ cup honey

4 tablespoons unsalted butter or ghee, softened or melted

1. Preheat your oven to 350°F/175°C.

2. Prepare a baking sheet with parchment paper or a nonstick baking mat.

3. Add the flour, salt, baking soda, cinnamon, ginger, and cloves to a large bowl and blend well.

4. Add the honey and butter to the dry ingredients and blend well until a soft dough forms.

5. Transfer the dough to the baking sheet and shape into a long log shape. I use the parchment paper to roll the dough.

6. Bake the log for 20 minutes, or until it is lightly browned. Remove from the oven and reduce the heat to 300°F/150°C.

7. Cool the log for about 10 minutes and then slice it into ½-inch-thick cookies. Place the cookie slices on their side on the baking sheet.

8. Place the biscotti back in the oven for 15 minutes. Take them out again, flip the biscotti over to the other side, and then place them back in the oven for another 15 minutes until they are fully crisped.

9. Cool the biscotti for at least 30 minutes.

10. Store in a dry, sealed container.

Nutrition per biscotto: *130 calories, 9 g fat, 12 g carbohydrate, 1 g fiber, 3 g protein*

French Vanilla Ice Cream

I love ice cream, and it's one of the best reasons for making dairy-free milk. It's naturally sweet, so it doesn't take much to sweeten it up and flavor it with honey or dates and some vanilla. There are a couple of ways to thicken ice cream made with dairy-free milk. I prefer using egg yolks; you can save the egg whites in the refrigerator for at least a week to use in other recipes.

Makes 4 servings or 1 quart

4 cups unsweetened almond milk

2 vanilla beans or 2 tablespoons vanilla extract

4 tablespoons honey, or to taste

6 egg yolks

1. Pour the milk into a saucepan and place over low to medium heat.

2. If you're using vanilla beans, slice them the long way and run the edge of the knife down the inside of the bean to scrape the seeds into the milk. If you're using vanilla extract, add it to the milk.

3. Stir the honey into the milk. Add the egg yolks and stir on and off to blend them with the milk. Heat slowly until the milk has thickened a bit and a light film of custard forms on the back of the stirring spoon.

4. Remove the mixture from the heat and let cool for at least 30 minutes at room temperature. Then cover and place in the refrigerator for at least 1 hour to chill. The longer the milk chills, the easier it will be to make the ice cream.

5. Pour the chilled mixture into an ice cream maker and follow the manufacturer's directions. (See the Quick Tip below if you don't have an ice cream maker.)

6. Store your ice cream in a sealed container in the freezer for up to a few weeks. The ice cream will get firmer as time goes by, so you may need to leave the container out at room temperature for several minutes before scooping.

Nutrition per serving: *277 calories, 9 g fat, 19 g carbohydrate, 1 g fiber, 5 g protein*

Quick Tip

◆ If you don't have an ice cream maker, place the ice cream in a blender container and chill in the freezer. Every half hour or so, take out the blender and blend the ice cream. Do this for several hours, or until it is the consistency that you want. Freeze in a sealed container.

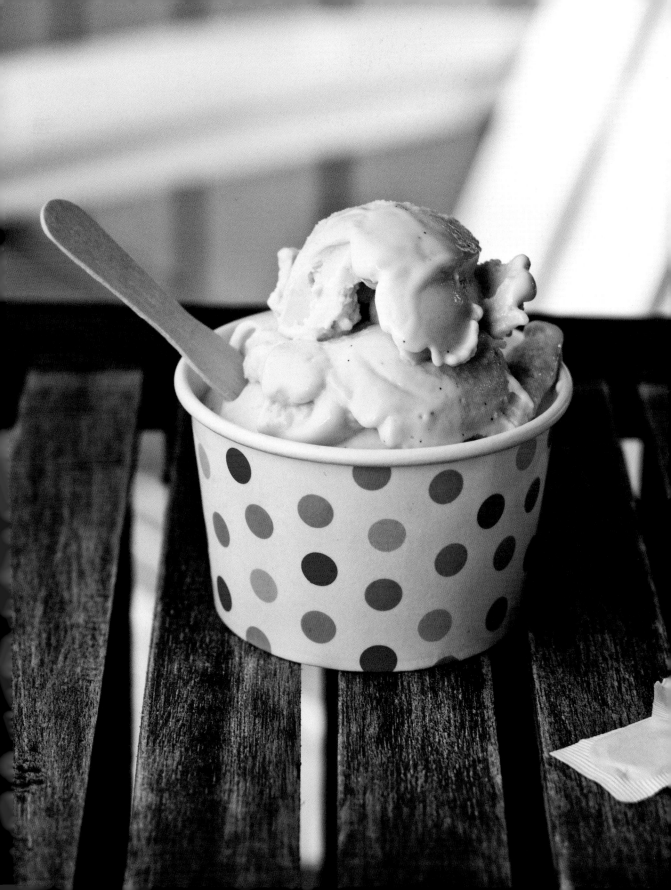

Apricot Frozen Yogurt

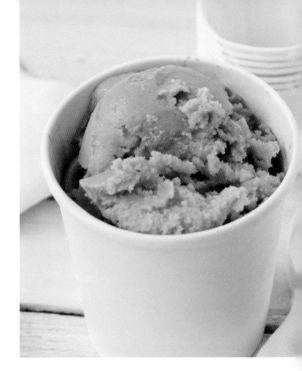

This frozen treat tastes exactly like a creamy sorbet, and there's no detectable sourness that yogurt sometimes imparts in ice cream recipes. I think it's the apricots dominating the flavor and successfully blending with the simple list of ingredients.

This yogurt goes perfectly between a couple of cookies to make a frozen yogurt sandwich—though the truth is, I eat it straight out of the container on warm summer months. If it's not summer, feel free to use frozen apricots, or if you don't have apricots, use fresh ripe peaches.

Makes 3 servings

8 ripe apricots (about 10 ounces), pits removed (or use frozen apricots)

½ cup honey

1 teaspoon fresh lemon juice

2 cups SCD Yogurt (page 20)

Blend all the ingredients together in a high-speed blender. Seal and store in the freezer for up to several weeks.

> **Nutrition per serving:** *277 calories, 0 g fat, 68 g carbohydrate, 2 g fiber, 5 g protein*

Avoid Sweet Overload

It's tempting to fill up on baked goods and honey-sweetened food, but avoid doing so. Instead, focus on making meals and healthy small plates and snacks, not treats and desserts. While you do need sugar, let it be a small part of a bigger meal and daily intake.

Waffle Cones

You'll need a waffle cone maker to make these, but if you're a fan like I am, it's worth the purchase and extra shelf space taken up by this gadget.

Makes 8 waffle cones

⅔ cup blanched almond flour

¼ teaspoon salt

2 large eggs

2 tablespoons honey

2 tablespoons unsalted butter, melted

1 teaspoon vanilla extract

1. Preheat your waffle cone maker per the manufacturer's directions.

2. Add the flour and salt to a bowl and whisk to blend.

3. Add the eggs, honey, butter, and vanilla, and whisk to combine.

4. Add 1 to 2 tablespoons batter to the waffle cone maker and close the lid.

5. When ready, take the flat waffle out. Use a dishcloth or napkin to hold the waffle when it first comes out because it is hot! Then immediately roll it using a cone roller.

6. Cool for a few minutes. Store in a sealed container.

> **Nutrition per waffle cone:** *114 calories, 9 g fat, 6 g carbohydrate, 1 g fiber, 4 g protein*

Cone-Making Tips

♦ As soon as you take the hot, flat waffle off the machine, place the cone roller on the waffle and extend the waffle a little bit beyond the bottom of the cone roller so you can close off the bottom.

♦ If you live in a humid climate, the cones will likely lose their crunch in a day or so. To regain the crunch, place the cones in a dehydrator, or warm oven no higher than 150°F/65°C, for about 10 minutes.

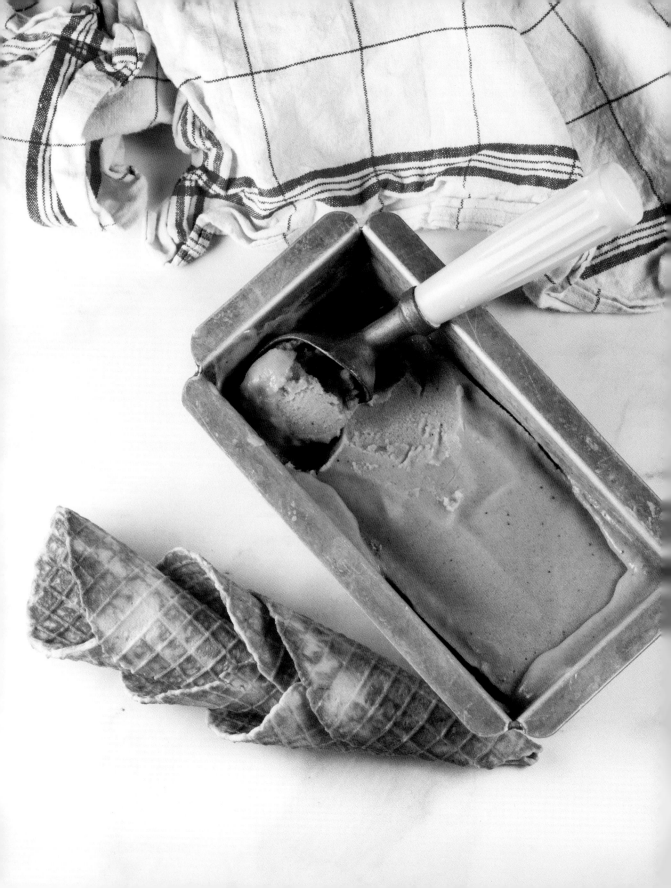

Pumpkin Ice Cream

Let me first say that you don't need to churn this ice cream. But you do have to freeze some bananas and pumpkin puree ahead of time.

Makes 4 servings

1 cup frozen Roasted Butternut Squash (page 130) or pumpkin puree

2 frozen bananas

½ cup coconut milk or other dairy-free milk

1 teaspoon pumpkin pie spice or ground cinnamon

1 teaspoon vanilla extract (optional)

1. Let the frozen squash puree and frozen bananas sit at room temperature for 10 minutes to soften a bit.

2. Place all the ingredients in a food processor or high-speed blender. Pulse until creamy, about a minute or so.

3. Serve immediately as soft-serve ice cream, or freeze for later. Defrost for at least 10 minutes once it is frozen.

> **Nutrition per serving:** *97 calories, 1 g fat, 21 g carbohydrate, 3 g fiber, 2 g protein*

Tips

♦ When I know I want to make this ice cream, I roast a large butternut squash and then freeze the puree in ice cube trays. Six frozen cubes are about 1 cup of pumpkin puree.

♦ Before freezing the bananas, peel and break into 2 or 4 pieces so they're easier to use in the food processor or blender later.

Banana "Ice Cream"

This banana ice cream has just one ingredient—bananas. It's so easy to make and naturally sweet. Just make sure, as with all SCD recipes, that you're using bananas that are fully ripe and have brown spots on them. This is because most of the carbohydrate in an unripe banana is in the form of starch. During the ripening process, the starch is converted to sugars that can more easily be digested and absorbed.

Makes 2 cups

4 medium ripe bananas, sliced into coins or large chunks

1. Freeze the banana pieces in an airtight container for at least 2 hours.

2. When you are ready to make the ice cream, place the frozen banana pieces in a blender or food processor.

3. Blend on high until creamy.

4. Consume immediately, store in a sealed container in the freezer, or add to ice pop molds.

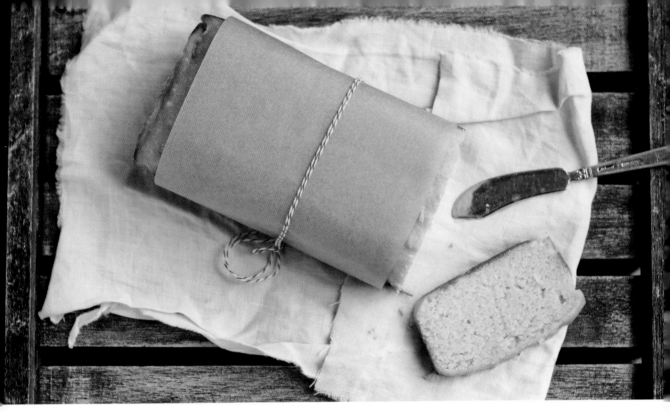

Lemon Pound Cake

This petite pound cake is a piece of cake heaven. I've wanted a pound cake recipe for myself for a long time, so this was the first sweet recipe I developed for this book.

The lemon in the cake provides a subtle tangy flavor, just as you'd expect. To get a stronger lemon flavor, you can add ½ teaspoon or so more lemon juice, which I sometimes do. If you don't have a citrus zester, you can use a cheese grater. Or use a vegetable peeler to peel the yellow skin off the lemon in very thin strips and then chop it as fine as possible.

Makes 8 servings

½ cup blanched almond flour

¼ cup coconut flour

½ teaspoon sea salt

4 eggs

¼ cup unsalted butter, melted

⅓ cup honey

¼ cup SCD Yogurt (page 20) or dairy-free milk

1 tablespoon fresh lemon juice

1 tablespoon fresh grated lemon zest (from 1 small lemon)

1 teaspoon vanilla extract

1. Preheat your oven to 325°F/165°C. Grease a loaf pan and/or line the bottom with parchment paper to make the cake easier to remove. (I usually do both for this recipe.) I use a 3½ x 7½-inch loaf pan, but a slightly larger one will work, too.

2. Blend the almond flour, coconut flour, and salt together in a bowl, either using an electric mixer or by hand.

3. Add the eggs, melted butter, honey, yogurt, lemon juice, zest, and vanilla extract and blend well, until all the lumps are gone.

4. Pour the batter into the prepared pan and bake for 50 minutes, or until a toothpick inserted in the center comes out clean.

5. Cool for 15 minutes or so and then serve. Store covered for a few days, or in the refrigerator for a few weeks.

Nutrition per serving: *140 calories, 10 g fat, 11 g carbohydrate, 2 g fiber, 5 g protein*

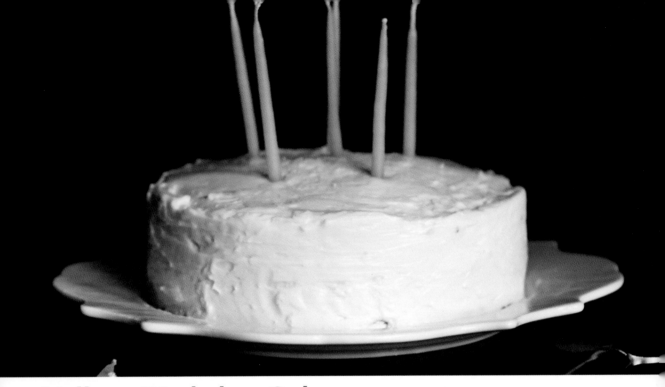

Yellow Birthday Cake

Almond and coconut flours are combined in this simple layer cake to give you the best of both worlds. A light, spongy cake that soaks up sweetness around it, it's a nice alternative to yellow cake made with just almond flour. This cake works well as a celebratory cake with frosting or other toppings. I don't make this as sweet as some might like. If you find you want it sweeter, replace some of the almond milk with honey, since this cake is plenty moist already.

This recipe is for a single cake layer, baked in an 8-inch round pan. To make a 2-layer cake, double the recipe and split the batter between two 8-inch cake pans. To make cupcakes, place nonstick muffin liners in a muffin tin and fill each liner about ⅔ full with batter. Bake for about 10 minutes, or until a toothpick inserted in the center of the cupcake comes out clean.

Makes 8 servings

½ cup blanched almond flour

¼ cup coconut flour

¼ teaspoon salt

¼ teaspoon baking soda

3 eggs

¼ cup unsalted butter or ghee (page 23), melted, or cooking oil

3 tablespoons honey

½ cup almond milk (or other dairy-free milk)

1 teaspoon vanilla extract

1. Preheat your oven to 325°F/165°C. Line the bottom of an 8-inch round cake pan with a parchment paper circle or other nonstick covering, or grease the pan well.

2. Blend the almond and coconut flours, salt, and baking soda in a mixing bowl. Add all the remaining ingredients and blend well. I use an electric mixer for this.

3. Pour the batter into the prepared pan and bake for 20 minutes, or until a toothpick inserted in the center of the cake comes out clean.

4. Let the cake cool on a wire rack for about 15 minutes, or an hour if you plan to frost the cake. Gently run a knife around the outside edge of the cake to make it easy to remove.

5. Once completely cooled, store covered at room temperature for a week or so, or store it in the refrigerator for a few weeks.

Nutrition per serving: *162 calories, 12 g fat, 10 g carbohydrate, 1 g fiber, 4 g protein*

Vanilla Cupcakes

I love simple recipes, and this one certainly falls into that category. It's also nut-free, and can be used to make a layer cake as well. To make a 2-layer cake, double the recipe and split it between 2 (8-inch) round baking pans. You can also substitute the oil in the recipe with butter, coconut oil, or shortening.

Makes 8 cupcakes

½ cup coconut flour

¼ teaspoon baking soda

¼ teaspoon salt

4 large eggs

⅓ cup olive oil

½ cup honey

2 tablespoons coconut milk or other dairy-free milk

1 tablespoon vanilla extract

1. Preheat the oven to 350°F/175°C.

2. Prepare a muffin tin with 8 cupcake liners.

3. Combine all the dry ingredients in a bowl and blend well.

4. Add the wet ingredients to the dry ingredients and use a mixer or spoon to blend well. Feel free to pulse the mixture in a food processor or blender to mix the batter.

5. Fill each cupcake liner about ¾ way with batter.

6. Bake for 20 minutes or until a toothpick inserted in the center of a cupcake comes out clean.

7. Cool and frost. Store covered in the refrigerator for a few weeks or freeze for a few months.

Nutrition per cupcake (unfrosted): *214 calories, 12 g fat, 22 g carbohydrate, 3 g fiber, 4 g protein*

Vanilla Donuts

Here's a simple vanilla donut recipe. It's lighter than those made with almond flour thanks to the coconut flour and lemon juice, which react with the baking soda to help them rise when baking.

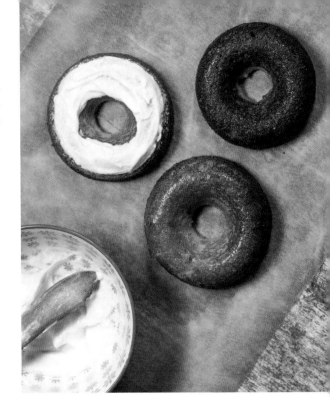

Makes 8 donuts

½ cup coconut flour

¼ teaspoon salt

¼ teaspoon baking soda

6 eggs

½ cup honey

1 tablespoon vanilla extract

½ cup unsalted butter, melted

1. Preheat your oven to 350°F/175°C.

2. Blend all the ingredients in a food processor or blender. You can also blend it by hand with a spoon.

3. Fill the donut pan circles about two-thirds of the way with batter.

4. Bake for 20 minutes, or until a toothpick inserted in the center of a donut comes out clean.

5. Store in the refrigerator for a week or so, or freeze for a few months.

Nutrition per donut: *254 calories, 6 g fat, 22 g carbohydrate, 3 g fiber, 6 g protein*

Tips

♦ Add ¼ cup blueberries for blueberry vanilla donuts; also add 1 tablespoon lemon juice for lemon blueberry donuts.

♦ I use Wilton's nonstick donut pan to make donuts but you can also use a silicon mold.

♦ To make this dairy-free, substitute oil for butter.

"Oatmeal" Raisin Cookies

If you don't have the time or patience to make these as whoopie pies, you can just make the oatmeal raisin cookies and be quite happy. While there's not actually any oatmeal in this recipe, the texture will please those who love oatmeal raisin cookies. And since these are soft and chewy, they make fine ice cream sandwiches (use the French Vanilla Ice Cream on page 186).

Watch the baking time, since these cookies brown on the bottom first. If you want a drier cookie, you can go a few minutes longer, but I like them moist with a bit of chewiness.

Makes 24 cookies

1 cup smooth roasted almond butter	2 teaspoons ground cinnamon
⅓ cup honey	½ teaspoon baking soda
1 egg	½ teaspoon salt
2 teaspoons vanilla extract	¾ cup raisins
½ cup unsweetened shredded coconut	Vanilla Frosting (page 205)

1. Preheat your oven to 350°F/175°C. Line a baking sheet with parchment paper or a nonstick baking mat.

2. Blend all the wet ingredients together using a spatula or a mixer, until creamy.

3. Combine the dry ingredients in a separate small bowl. Add them to the almond butter mixture and blend well.

4. Spoon about 1 tablespoon of batter per cookie onto the prepared baking sheet, spacing the cookies about 1 inch apart. If you prefer a flatter cookie/pie, flatten the cookies a bit with the bottom of a glass jar, spoon, or spatula.

5. Bake for 10 to 12 minutes, or until the edges are just starting to brown.

6. Transfer the cookies to a wire rack to cool. Make whoopie pies by sandwiching pairs of cookies together with vanilla frosting filling in the middle. Store the cookies covered at room temperature for about a week, or in the refrigerator for a few weeks.

Nutrition per cookie: *129 calories, 8 g fat, 15 g carbohydrate, 2 g fiber, 3 g protein*

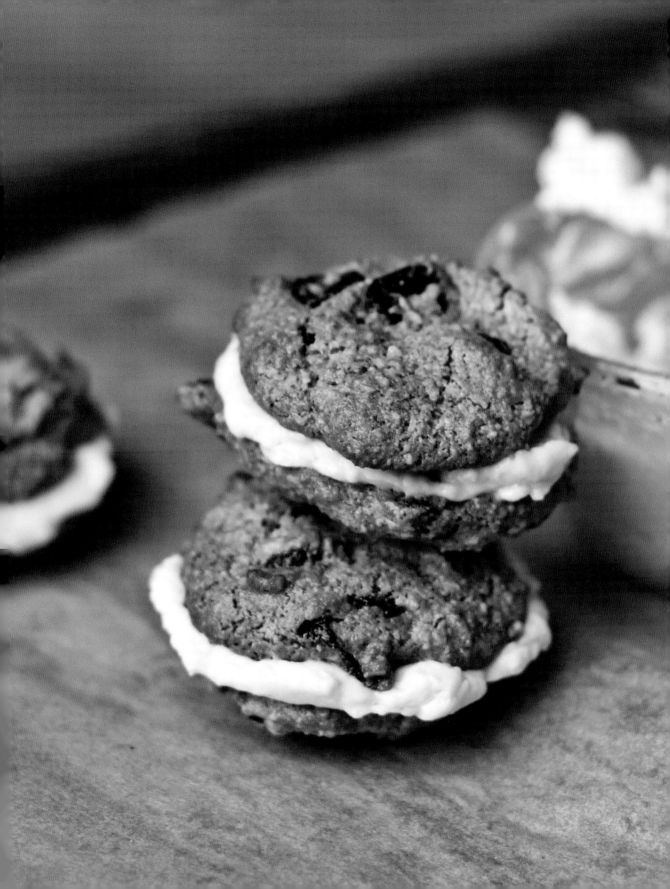

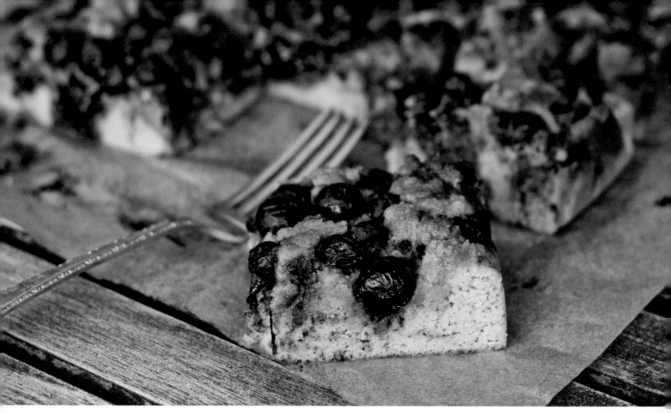

Blueberry Cinnamon Coffee Cake

Okay, there's no coffee in this recipe, but you can certainly pair it with all kinds of beverages—and with ice cream, of course. It's a friendly cake, meant for sharing after a meal or maybe when relaxing on a lazy Sunday morning.

Feel free to switch berries if something else is in season. I tend to use frozen berries when it's not blueberry season, just because I love the way blueberries and cinnamon work together. Don't be put off by the long list of layers and ingredients—a lot of it is the same kind of ingredient, and each layer comes together quite easily. If you want to forgo a layer, I'd say that the cake will taste good even without the crumble topping, though the crumble completes this quintessential cake.

I've arranged this recipe in the order of the layers that go into your baking pan. The recipe fills an 8 x 8-inch or smaller pan. The batter may seem a bit skimpy, but it does rise a bit, and the layers add to the cake's height.

Makes 9 squares

CAKE LAYER

½ cup blanched almond flour

¼ cup coconut flour

¼ teaspoon salt

¼ teaspoon baking soda

½ teaspoon ground cinnamon

3 eggs

¼ cup unsalted butter, melted

3 tablespoons honey

1 teaspoon vanilla extract

½ cup almond milk (or other dairy-free milk or SCD Yogurt, page 20)

CRUMBLE LAYER

1 teaspoon ground cinnamon

⅛ teaspoon baking soda

¼ teaspoon salt

1 cup blanched almond flour (or other nut flour)

2 tablespoons honey

1 tablespoon unsalted butter, softened

¼ cup crushed walnuts (optional)

BLUEBERRY LAYER

1 cup blueberries (fresh or frozen)

1. Preheat your oven to 350°F/175°C.

2. Line the bottom of an 8-inch square (or smaller) baking pan with parchment paper.

3. For the cake layer, combine the almond flour, coconut flour, salt, baking soda, and cinnamon in a mixing bowl; blend well.

4. Add the eggs, butter, honey, vanilla, and almond milk. Mix until well blended; I use an electric stand mixer for this step.

5. Scoop the cake batter into the prepared pan and shuffle the pan to spread the batter evenly.

6. In another bowl, combine all the crumble layer ingredients and blend with a fork until crumbly. Spread evenly over the top of the cake layer.

7. Spread the blueberries across the top of the crumble layer.

8. Bake for 40 minutes, or until the top is browned and a toothpick inserted in the center comes out clean.

9. Let cool, slice, and serve. You can store the cake at room temperature, covered, for a few days or in the refrigerator for a few weeks.

Nutrition per square: *192 calories, 13 g fat, 16 g carbohydrate, 2 g fiber, 4 g protein*

Quick Tip

◆ If you really like cinnamon, you can double the recipe for the cinnamon layer. And if you like nuts, add ¼ cup finely chopped walnuts to the crumble layer to add a bit of a crunch.

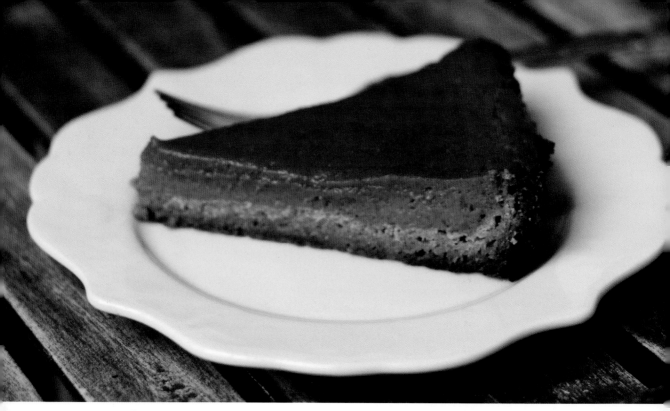

Pumpkin Pie

This is a classic pumpkin pie that happens to be dairy-free. If you don't feel like whipping up a crust, the pumpkin filling tastes good baked on its own, without a crust—it's kind of like pumpkin custard.

As for the baking time, it will depend on the size of your pie pan. The custard filling will bake faster in a large, flat tart pan than in a deep pie dish. Because my tart pan isn't nonstick, I line the bottom with parchment paper. You can also grease the sides a bit.

Makes 8 servings

CRUST

2 cups blanched almond flour

¼ teaspoon salt

¼ teaspoon baking soda

½ teaspoon ground cinnamon

¼ cup coconut oil, unsalted butter, or ghee (page 23)

1 teaspoon vanilla extract

1 tablespoon honey

FILLING

1¾ cups (about 15 ounces) canned pumpkin puree or roasted squash (page 130; butternut squash is the best)

¼ cup dairy-free milk (coconut or almond, or substitute more squash instead)

3 eggs

½ cup honey (or a bit more, depending on the sweetness of the squash or pumpkin)

1 tablespoon vanilla extract

½ teaspoon salt

1 teaspoon ground cinnamon

½ teaspoon ground nutmeg

¼ teaspoon each ground ginger, ground cloves, ground allspice, and ground cardamom (optional, for a spicier pie)

1. Preheat your oven to 350°F/175°C.

2. To make the crust, place the almond flour, salt, baking soda, and cinnamon in the bowl of a food processor and pulse briefly to blend. Add the coconut oil, vanilla, and honey and process briefly so that you have small grains of dough that stick together when you press them with your fingers.

3. Press the crust into a 8 or 9-inch pie pan or tart pan using your fingers. Line with parchment paper and fill with pie weights (or dried beans), or insert a toothpick in several places around the crust, to keep the crust from bubbling while it browns. Bake for 5 minutes, or until the crust is slightly browned.

4. Let the crust cool for 10 minutes and then place it in the freezer for about 15 minutes.

5. Meanwhile, combine all the pie filling ingredients in a bowl, whisking to blend well.

6. Pour the filling into the chilled crust. I like to pour it right up to the edge of the crust to keep the crust from getting too brown. You can also cover the crust edges with foil to prevent them from browning too fast.

7. Bake for about 35 minutes if you're using a tart pan, or until the outer edges of the filling are firm. A deeper pie pan will take closer to 45 minutes.

8. Let cool for at least 30 minutes before slicing into 8 pieces. Store the pie in the refrigerator, covered, for up to a week or so.

> **Nutrition per serving:** *220 calories, 5 g fat, 26 g carbohydrate, 2 g fiber, 5 g protein*

Breakfast Cookies

I'm about to give you a good excuse to eat cookies for breakfast, or any other time of day. Pack a cookie with enough protein and vitamins, and you have yourself a respectable breakfast treat.

Another thing I like about these packets of nutritional power is that they can easily be customized to your own taste. Your favorite nuts, seeds, and dried fruit will all work in this recipe. It's that easy. One of my readers leaves the honey out and says that these cookies still taste great.

Makes 24 cookies

2½ cups blanched almond flour (or almond meal or other nut flour)

½ teaspoon salt

½ teaspoon baking soda

½ cup unsalted butter, coconut oil, or ghee (page 23), melted

½ cup honey

1 egg

1 tablespoon vanilla extract

2 cups nuts, dried fruit, and/or seeds (or anything else your heart desires)

1. Preheat your oven to 350°F/175°C.

2. Combine the almond flour, salt, and baking soda in a bowl and blend, using a whisk or fork.

3. Add the remaining ingredients and combine well, stirring with a fork or spoon. If the batter is a bit too soft to handle, place it in the freezer for 5 minutes.

4. Drop tablespoons of batter onto the baking sheets, spacing them about 1 inch apart.

5. Bake for 12 to 15 minutes, or until the cookies are starting to brown around the edges. (If you prefer your cookies slightly crunchier, turn off the oven and leave them in for another 15 minutes or so; or place them in a dehydrator on a fairly low temperature for about 30 minutes.)

6. Store the cookies in a sealed container at room temperature for a few days, in the refrigerator for a few weeks, or in the freezer for a few months.

Nutrition per cookie: *226 calories, 10 g fat, 35 g carbohydrate, 2 g fiber, 4 g protein*

Vanilla Frosting

For most of my family, a celebration isn't complete until we have a yellow cake with frosting. But any cake you like can be a birthday cake. It could be banana bread drizzled with white glaze and candied nuts. Or it could be a tower of your favorite pancakes, with cream and berries between the layers and syrup drizzled over the top. Or it might be fresh berries between cake layers, topped with whipped crème frâiche. For a flavor twist, you can add a little cinnamon and nutmeg to this dairy-free vanilla frosting.

If you're craving the familiar, though, bake two layers of yellow cake (page 194), let them cool, and make this or one of the following frostings. Be sure to wait to frost your cake until it's completely cool—otherwise the frosting will melt. Then spread on a thin layer of frosting to seal the crumbs. Chill the cake for 10 minutes and then finish frosting it.

Makes 8 (1½-tablespoon) servings

½ cup Spectrum shortening (see Product Sources, page 214)

¼ cup honey

½ teaspoon vanilla extract (or vanilla bean seeds)

1 tablespoon almond milk (or other dairy-free milk), or more if needed to soften the frosting and add flavor

Using an electric mixer, blend all the ingredients together until you have the consistency of a creamy frosting. Feel free to adjust the sweetness and the amount of milk to get the consistency and flavor you prefer. Use this frosting at room temperature.

Nutrition per serving: *163 calories, 14 g fat, 9 g carbohydrate, 0 g fiber, 0 g protein*

Marshmallow Meringue Frosting

This combination of egg whites and honey, with a few intricately timed steps, will yield you a shiny, light meringue frosting. Lemon juice or vinegar helps the frosting stay fluffy, and a little bit of vanilla adds flavor.

Makes 8 (½-cup) servings

¼ cup honey

2 egg whites

¼ teaspoon fresh lemon juice or white vinegar (optional)

¼ teaspoon vanilla extract (optional)

1. In a small saucepan over low to medium heat, bring the honey to a steady low boil. Boil for about 5 to 10 minutes, or until the honey starts to darken. It's ready when you drop some in cold water and it forms a small ball.

2. Add the egg whites and lemon juice to a bowl. Whisk the egg whites in a mixer with a whisk attachment, or by hand, until they form stiff peaks and have a glossy finish. While you're whipping the egg whites, slowly drizzle in the honey and the vanilla. If you're using a mixer, the honey may spray a bit, so try to drizzle it down the side of the bowl, away from the whisk.

3. Use this frosting soon, as it tends to deflate a bit as it absorbs moisture from the air. You can store it in the refrigerator for about a week, covered, and rewhip it if it begins to separate.

> **Nutrition per serving:** *45 calories, 0 g fat, 9 g carbohydrate, 0 g fiber, 1 g protein*

Cream Cheese Frosting

This is a simple topping that goes great on muffins and cakes or as a tasty dip for sliced fruit. The recipe makes enough to frost a few muffins or to use as dip. Double or triple these amounts if you're frosting a cake.

Makes 4 (2-tablespoon) servings

½ cup Dripped SCD Yogurt (page 21) or farmer's cheese

½ teaspoon honey

Combine the yogurt and honey in a bowl, blending well. Chill until ready to use. Depending on the thickness of your yogurt, you may want to bring this frosting to room temperature before spreading it on a cake or cupcakes.

> **Nutrition per serving:** *15 calories, 0 g fat, 2 g carbohydrate, 0 g fiber, 2 g protein*

Vanilla Buttercream Frosting

When you need a simple, vanilla buttercream frosting, this is it. Use a light-colored honey to get it as close to white as possible. Mixing it well will help with turning it white as well. This recipe will frost 8 cupcakes or 1 layer cake.

Makes 8 (2-tablespoon) servings

½ cup unsalted butter, softened

½ cup light-colored honey

2 teaspoons vanilla extract

1. Add all the ingredients to a bowl of a standing mixer with a flat mixing attachment, or use a hand mixer or food processor.

2. Mix on a low speed until the butter starts to soften.

3. Increase the speed until the butter is creamy and lightens in color, about a minute or so.

4. Store in the refrigerator for a few weeks, and bring to room temperature for 30 minutes or so before using.

> **Nutrition per serving:** *271 calories, 23 g fat, 18 g carbohydrate, 0 g fiber, 0 g protein*

Strawberry Buttercream Frosting

Here's a fun take on the Vanilla Buttercream Frosting recipe above. You can use fresh or freeze-dried strawberries. If you use fresh, first mash into a puree (or puree them in a food processor or blender).

Makes 8 (2-tablespoon) servings

½ cup unsalted butter, softened

½ cup light-colored honey

2 teaspoons vanilla extract

¼ cup freeze-dried or pureed strawberries

1. Add all the ingredients to a bowl of a standing mixer with a flat mixing attachment, or use a hand mixer or food processor.

2. Mix on a low speed until the butter starts to soften.

3. Increase the speed until the butter is creamy and lightens in color, about a minute or so.

4. Store in the refrigerator for a few weeks, and bring to room temperature for 30 minutes or so before using.

> **Nutrition per serving:** *273 calories, 23 g fat, 18 g carbohydrate, 0 g fiber, 0 g protein*

Lemon Cream Frosting

Lemon and a creamy foundation make for a great base for making a tangy frosting. There are 2 frostings here: one using coconut cream and the other using yogurt. You can use any yogurt you prefer, either dairy-based or dairy-free.

Makes 8 (1-tablespoon) servings

¼ cup thick yogurt

1 teaspoon lemon juice

3 teaspoons honey

¼ teaspoon vanilla extract

Add all the ingredients to a bowl of a standing mixer with a flat mixing attachment, or use a hand mixer or food processor. Mix until creamy and well blended.

Nutrition per serving: 39 calories, 1 g fat, 8 g carbohydrate, 0 g fiber, 1 g protein

Tip

◆ You can obtain coconut cream by refrigerating a container of full-fat coconut milk overnight. The cream rises to the top and can be easily removed with a spoon. Another way to obtain coconut cream is to process the fresh white meat of a coconut until it is soft and creamy.

White Glaze

Makes 8 (1-tablespoon) servings

½ cup coconut butter (see Product Sources, page 214)

½ tablespoon honey

¼ teaspoon vanilla extract

1. Place the coconut butter and honey in a small, heatproof bowl.

2. Immerse the bowl halfway in another bowl or a saucepan containing hot water, or place it in a warm oven, until the butter is soft but not fully melted.

3. Add the vanilla and stir until everything is well blended. Drizzle over your cake.

Nutrition per serving: 125 calories, 14 g fat, 1 g carbohydrate, 0 g fiber, 0 g protein

Measurements and Substitutions

Common Equivalents

1 gallon = 4 quarts = 8 pints = 16 cups = 128 fluid ounces = 3.8 liters

1 quart = 2 pints = 4 cups = 32 ounces = .95 liter

1 pint = 2 cups = 16 ounces = 480 ml

1 cup = 8 ounces = 240 ml

¼ cup = 4 tablespoons = 12 teaspoons = 2 ounces = 60 ml

1 tablespoon = 3 teaspoons = ½ ounce = 15 ml

Temperature Conversions

Fahrenheit (°F)	Celsius (°C)	Gas Mark
200°F	95°C	0
225°F	110°C	¼
250°F	120°C	½
275°F	135°C	1
300°F	150°C	2
325°F	165°C	3
350°F	175°C	4
375°F	190°C	5
400°F	200°C	6
425°F	220°C	7
450°F	230°C	8
475°F	245°C	9

Volume Conversions

U.S.	U.S.	Metric
1 tablespoon (3 teaspoons)	½ fluid ounce	15 ml
¼ cup	2 fluid ounces	60 ml
⅓ cup	3 fluid ounces	90 ml
½ cup	4 fluid ounces	120 ml
⅔ cup	5 fluid ounces	150 ml
¾ cup	6 fluid ounces	180 ml
1 cup	8 fluid ounces	240 ml
2 cups	16 fluid ounces	480 ml

Weight

U.S.	Metric
½ ounce	15 grams
1 ounce	30 grams
2 ounces	60 grams
¼ pound	115 grams
⅓ pound	150 grams
½ pound	225 grams
¾ pound	350 grams
1 pound	450 grams

Common Ingredient Equivalents

Almond flour ½ cup = 48 g	Coconut flour ¼ cup = 26 g
Honey ¼ cup = 85 g	Butter ½ cup = 8 tablespoons
Olive oil ¼ cup = 2 ounces	Coconut oil ¼ cup = 52 g

Ingredient Substitutions

Here are some suggested substitutions for a few commonly used ingredients. Substituting ingredients successfully can vary from recipe to recipe—you'll want to take into account how swapping out one ingredient for another will affect the overall taste and texture of a dish.

Baking Powder

Baking powder is avoided on the SCD because it contains starch or other caking additives. It's quite easy to substitute baking soda and another component instead:

1 teaspoon baking powder = ½ teaspoon baking soda + ½ teaspoon lemon juice

1 teaspoon baking powder = ½ teaspoon baking soda + ½ teaspoon plain yogurt

Eggs

The egg is a tricky ingredient to swap out because it's a flavorless binding agent. Eggs can be replicated somewhat with the alternatives below. Keep in mind that banana has a distinct flavor, so use it when you want that flavor. Applesauce not only acts as a binding agent and adds sweetness, but it can also be used as a substitute for oil or butter by adding moisture and volume. Pureed prunes (baby food), like applesauce, bind and add sweetness.

¼ cup mashed banana = 1 egg

¼ cup unsweetened applesauce = 1 egg

3 tablespoons pureed prunes = 1 egg

Baking soda plus vinegar can also be used to replace eggs. Add the baking soda to the dry ingredients in the recipe and add the vinegar to the wet ingredients, then combine the dry and wet ingredients. A chemical reaction will release gas and lift your batter. Place the batter in the oven as soon as you combine the dry and wet ingredients, before the gas can escape.

1 teaspoon baking soda + 1 teaspoon apple cider vinegar = 1 egg

Yogurt, both dairy and dairy-free, binds and adds moisture.

¼ cup of yogurt = 1 egg

Duck Eggs

For people who can better digest duck eggs than chicken eggs, you can replace duck eggs in recipes calling for eggs.

1 duck egg = 1 chicken egg

Honey

Dates are an excellent sweetener alternative to honey. My favorite date is the Medjool, but others work, too.

¼ cup honey = ¼ cup chopped dates

Nut Butter

While the flavor may change a bit, in general you can replace any nut butter with a seed butter, such as sunflower seed or sesame seed butter (tahini).

nut butter = seed butter

Vanilla

Both the shells and the seeds of vanilla beans contain vanilla flavoring. To use the seeds in place of extract, choose a soft, fresh bean (not dried out), slice it down the middle the long way, and then use the edge of the knife to scrape out the seeds. Here's an easy equivalent for swapping the seeds for vanilla extract:

seeds from 1 vanilla bean = 1 tablespoon vanilla extract

Resources

Books

Gottschall, Elaine Gloria. *Breaking the Vicious Cycle: Intestinal Health Through Diet*. Baltimore, ON: The Kirkton Press, 1994.

Websites

Comfy Belly	comfybelly.com
Breaking the Vicious Cycle	breakingtheviciouscycle.info/home
The Gottschall Autism Center	gottschallcenter.com
Liberated Specialty Foods	liberatedspecialtyfoods.com
Pecan Bread (focus on children)	pecanbread.com
SCD Bakery	scdbakery.com
SCD Recipe	scdrecipe.com
Wellbee's	wellbees.com

Product Sources

Product	Source	Contact Info
Almond flour	Amazon	amazon.com
	Costco	costco.com
	Honeyville	honeyvillegrain.com
	Hughson Nut	hughsonnut.com
	Trader Joe's	traderjoes.com
	Wellbee's	wellbees.com
	Whole Foods	wholefoods.com
Baking papers, plastic	If You Care	ifyoucare.com
	Natural Value	naturalvalue.com
Dehydrator	Excalibur	excaliburdehydrator.com
Dried fruit and nuts	Nuts.com	nuts.com
	Eden Foods	edenfoods.com
Donuts and bagels	Wilton nonstick donut pans	wilton.com
	Wappa nonstick silicone molds	wappakitchen.net
Honey (Locally sourced brands are best, in general. Manuka honey comes from New Zealand or Australia.) Note: Children under the age of 1 year should not eat honey.	Trader Joe's	traderjoes.com
	Bee Raw Honey	beeraw.com
	Glory Bee (Oregon-based)	glorybeehoney.com
Probiotics	GI ProHealth	giprohealth.com
Vanilla, dried herbs, spices	Frontier	frontiercoop.com
	Simply Organic	simplyorganic.com
	Flavorganics	flavorganics.com
	Mountain Rose Herbs	mountainroseherbs.com
Vegetable shortening and high-heat oils	Spectrum	spectrumorganics.com
Vinegars and oils	Eden Foods	edenfoods.com
	Spectrum	spectrumorganics.com
Yogurt Starter	GI ProHealth	giprohealth.com

Recipe Index

Acknowledgments

To my boys, my family and friends, and Comfy Belly readers who inspire me every day.

And for the unwavering love and dedication of Elaine Gottschall and all parents, families, and friends of those whose lives have been challenged by health issues.

About the Author

Erica Kerwien is a writer and cookbook author. When one of her sons was diagnosed with Crohn's disease, she set out to help him restore his health in the best way possible—with food. Along the way, she discovered the Specific Carbohydrate Diet (SCD), which changed the way her family eats and cooks. Erica started the website *Comfy Belly* (comfybelly.com) to track and share her recipes, and it has become a valuable resource for recipes that are low-carb, gluten-free, refined sugar-free, lactose-free, dairy-free, and grain-free.

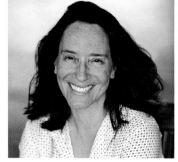

© Studio B Portraits